Maggie's
Food Strategy
Book

Books by Maggie Lettvin

THE BEAUTIFUL MACHINE

GUIDE TO FITNESS AFTER FIFTY

MAGGIE'S BACK BOOK:
Healing the Hurt in Your Lower Back

MAGGIE'S WOMAN'S BOOK:
Her Personal Plan for Health and Fitness
for Women of Every Age

MAGGIE'S FOOD STRATEGY BOOK:
Taking Charge of Your Diet for
Lifelong Health and Vitality

MAGGIE'S
Food Strategy
❧ BOOK ❧

*Taking Charge of Your Diet
for Lifelong Health and Vitality*

MAGGIE LETTVIN

❧

Foreword by
GEORGE PLOTKIN, Ph.D.

Houghton Mifflin Company • Boston 1987

Library of Congress Cataloging-in-Publication Data

Lettvin, Maggie.
Maggie's food strategy book.

Bibliography: p.
Includes index.
1. Low-calorie diet. 2. Nutrition. 3. Health.
4. Menus. 5. Food—Caloric content—Tables.
6. Food—Vitamin content—Tables. I. Title.
RM222.2.L428 1987 613.2'5 86-21396
ISBN 0-395-37983-0
ISBN 0-395-43098-4 (pbk.)

Printed in the United States of America

I 10 9 8 7 6 5 4 3 2 1

Book design by Victoria Hartman

To each of the men and women who
came through my classes at MIT
I still remember each of you
by your face and your problems.
Many of the answers to the problems
which we worked out then together,
with you specifically in mind,
are reflected in this book.
I hope you all are continuing to
seek health.

Acknowledgments

Thanks to Ruth Hapgood, my patient editor, who went over and over this manuscript. Ruth also led me to some new sources.

Thanks to Peggy L. Anderson, manuscript editor supreme. Would it ever have been finished without her?

Thanks again to Charlotte Michaelson, my friend and former assistant producer at WGBH-TV, who helped me arrange the meals and read and edited for me. This is our fourth book together.

Thanks to Penny Chase Williams for some last-minute typing. Our fourth book together.

Thanks to Leslie Brown for hours of typing. Our second book together.

Thanks to Suzanne Brown and Janice Novak, who read for me and who dug out virtually all the numbers in the food sources for me. Janice also helped with the typing and, most important, ran the nutrition programs for me when my own program failed to arrive. Third book with Suzanne, second with Janice.

George Plotkin was my nutrition expert. A biochemist with extensive learning and understanding, George was generous enough to read my book and to check it for facts. His foreword is a gem.

Jerry, my husband, always reads my work. His corrections are fewer with this book. I'm wearing him down.

Six readers?! I need all the help I can get.

Contents

Acknowledgments   vii
Foreword by George Plotkin, Ph.D.   xi
Introduction   xiii

Part I · The Art of Dieting: A New Look

1. You Are Unique   3
2. A Closer Look at What We Eat   16

Part II · Eight Diets

3. About the Eight Diets   33
4. The Sweet Diet   53
5. The Regularity Diet   69
6. The Raw Diet   89
7. The Shine (Anti-Stress) Diet   104
8. The Two-Minute Diet   125
9. The High-Protein, Low-Carbohydrate Diet   138
10. The Pocket Diet   157
11. The Lean, Clean Machine Diet   173

Part III · Balancing Food and Movement with the Cards

12. Eat — and Keep Moving   187
13. Changing Habits for a New Balance   203

Part IV · Making Your Diet Better and Better

14. "Add 'Em": The Choice Filler Foods, and More   225
15. "Chuck 'Em" — and Good Riddance!   252

Part V · Diet Master

16. Making It Work: Designing Your Food Strategy   273
17. Nutrient Needs, Nutrient Sources   288

Postscript   335
Bibliography   337
Index   339

Foreword

Food, like sex and shelter, has a wordless language of the most ancient order, whose grammar is specific to the area and the culture that speaks it. It is the language of survival, the maintenance of the present members of the culture as well as the guarantee of support for the future. Food has as its foundation a trinity — cultivation, storage, and preparation — each linked to the other, no one being sufficient to ensure survival.

The planting, herding, harvesting, storing, and cooking of food become the subjects of ritual, be it an ancient corn dance, a priestly blessing of the fishing fleet, or a blue-ribbon French chef making passes over the next entrée with just the right spice. Ritual is the timekeeper — when to plant, when to reap, when to serve. In the absence of ritual, a crop may not yield the food necessary for the community, a shoaling fish may elude the net, and an undercooked meal may sour the palate.

Details of the ritual are not incidental. Adding a mint leaf to a clutch of grain may seem a quaint custom, but it dissuades the mouse who might otherwise take up residence and spoil the harvest. Only later does mint, basil, or bay leaf acquire the role of a spice. Placing cayenne on cooking flesh discourages dogs, cats, and rats, and in so doing allows meal preparation to go on in the absence of the cook, who may be needed in the field. Pepper is now added to many foods, but for taste rather than to repel cats.

In the tropics of Southeast Asia, one is immediately aware of another pest, insects. Any cooking pot left uncovered would ordinarily swarm with flies. The mode of cooking, though, makes flies avoid the open kettles. The answer again comes from what we now call a spice, lemon grass, a plant possessing citraldehyde, anathema to insects (and used in the wonderful citronella candle) but unfortunately a potent cardiovascular corrupter of mammals. Why, then, doesn't the citraldehyde harm the villager? The answer is the high levels of vitamin A also found in lemon grass, which more than balances the action of citraldehyde. Lemon grass extract, devoid of or attenuated in vitamin A, is still highly toxic!

This last example brings us from ritual to recipe. Ritual provided a method to ensure safety and stability, and evolved over generations of trial and error. Recipe is what remains as curious incantations after the supposed purpose has vanished. But food, as I've said, is a language, personal as our own body chemistry, bearing the signatures of our ancestors. Therefore, to say a meal is a collection of protein, carbohydrate, and the like is to say an Auden poem is a collection of words — true, but far from sufficient.

Maggie Lettvin's volume is neither a diet book nor a cookbook. Agreed, it contains recipes, agreed it suggests diets. However, its purpose is to reacquaint you with a variety of languages and dialects that may remind you of what your family spoke a generation ago. It reestablishes a sense that food is a crucial part of your heritage and as such cannot be neglected. Taken as a beginner's grammar, it will prove more enduring than the dozens of generic diet volumes and cookbooks that, in all likelihood, litter your shelves.

George Plotkin, Ph.D.
Visiting Scientist
MIT Communications Physiology Laboratory

Introduction

I come from a family that is seriously interested in health-building. For several generations my mother's side of the family was convinced that proper food prevented illness. The dedication with which my mother applied herself to the task of giving us the best of everything even led her to buy a farm so that we could have our own raw milk, buttermilk, sweet butter, our own fresh vegetables, our own whole-grain cereals and bread, our own unsprayed apples, our own chickens, our own pigs. Nothing stopped her when it came to preserving our health and setting an example for us. I can remember how as a child I would watch my mother lying in our narrow upstairs hallway doing her daily exercises. Every summer she rose at five or six to get her housework done early, packed a lunch for the five of us and, with the weakest one in the wagon, walked us all three miles each way to the beach so that we got our exercise and sun every sunny summer's day. Her commitment was total. She is now over ninety, active, intelligent, has a wicked sense of humor, and is a joy to be around.

Though my mother was on excellent — even friendly — terms with all the doctors of Salem, New Jersey, she certainly used them only when absolutely necessary. She questioned them mercilessly about their intended treatment when one of us fell ill. She felt it was *her* responsibility to keep us healthy and took this responsibility to be a serious commitment that involved our entire lifestyle.

The emphasis was always to build and to maintain health. She was not really ahead of her time, for there was a small ground swell building up. (That was the time of John Harvey Kellogg, Horace Fletcher, Bernarr Macfadden, and others.) But my mother was certainly very committed to fighting actively to maintain health. And so, of course, it became imbedded in my mind that the true responsibility for your health lies within your own hands for the most part. That belief was among my mother's greatest gifts to me, along with common sense and compassion. Like all important gifts, they entail responsibility.

A number of years ago when I suffered a whiplash injury, I first took to my bed as I was directed, to allow the pain to abate. But when, after six months of more rest than I ever wanted, I was still not free of pain, I refused surgery but belatedly took an active part in my own recovery. I exercised very delicately, changed my diet to take care of the added stress, and only then became gradually totally free of pain. (Two years from the date of the accident.) It was not easy. It was not fast. It was not without some failures. But on the whole I slowly recovered my *self*.

All of this is to enlighten you as to my own views and to the suggestions that you will find within this book. *First of all you do everything that you can to improve yourself!* A good diagnosis from the best doctor you can find needs to be part of this strategy if you feel you may be ill or know that you are sick. If, on the other hand, you just feel that you could be healthier, the ways to improve your own lifestyle and health are wide open.

For years I have been observing a steady stream of people with a wide variety of symptoms — most often physical and related to diseases they have been suffering for anywhere from several weeks to a lifetime. Anyone engaged in trying to relieve distress sees some people who have a collection of very mild complaints and others with serious and even life-threatening conditions. Just consider everyday chronic problems: dizziness, overweight, premenstrual syndrome, broken blood vessels, ulcerated legs and feet, "busy legs," lymphedema (swelling of different parts of the body due to excessive lymph fluid being held by tissues), falling hair, acne, dermatitis, dry hair, splitting nails, extreme nervousness, depression, scaly skin, foul body odor, balance problems — the list goes on and on.

I never deal with any of these symptoms from a medical point of view. All my clients must be cleared through their doctors and advised by them before coming to me. My only role is to suggest ways for each individual to build up his or her own health as far as is possible so they can withstand the problems they suffer. Very often the symptoms and complaints are made much worse by neglect of the very factors that help us to withstand them: nutrition and practiced positioning and movement of the body. But the nutritional points are not easy to make. They are distributed over a wide range of professional textbooks. Throughout this book, I have tried to give you a short guide to professionally accepted notions about what constitutes good nutrition. In Chapters 14 and 17, in particular, you will find many lists of especially nutritious foods. The Bibliography cites the texts from which my information is taken, if you want to pursue your own study.

Since I have always strongly believed in good diet, I spend much time and effort researching each individual's problem from both a nutritional and a physiological point of view. It takes a little time to see what an interesting pursuit this can be. My early approach, which involved putting together explicit collections of nutrients to deal with individual symptoms, gave way finally to a general method designed to supply a nutrient-rich intake that would give each individual body all the raw materials needed to allow it to fight its own battles. In short, it seems better strategy simply to build general health in a straightforward manner by supplying the full complement of nutritional building blocks, rather than by shoring up the system here and there with special nutrients used for special effects.

It is easy to design a generally rich intake with a whole shelf of separate supplements but much harder to do with ordinary food, which at first seems surprising. But the way foods are grown, stored, transported, prepared, and so on often takes out nutrients that are originally plentiful. And then the ability of your particular civilized system to deal properly with breaking down the foods until they are of the proper consistency for digestion varies markedly from one person to another. So also does the absorption, storage, and rate of use.

My first, and very effective choice was to suggest supplements not in pill or capsule form, for the most part, but in powder form. Pills and capsules occasionally do not break up in the digestive tract, particularly in people with poor digestion, who most need the nutrients. Providing nutrients in powdered form to be added to liquids proved very successful. Little symptoms disappeared one by one, at first slowly, then at a faster rate; and finally an obvious return to much-improved health began to show itself — in those who could stomach my "witch's brew." No, *I did not cure disease!* No, if there was a disease, not *all* the symptoms would disappear. A good supply of nutrients simply allowed the body to help itself — to make itself healthier than it had been and to improve in ways only secondarily having to do with any disease condition.

When the body is under stress of any sort, whether emotional, caused by a sudden serious physical trauma, or by ongoing insults *that it does not have enough reserves to handle,* the result will be little discrepancies between the body's nutritional needs and its ability to fulfill them. The extra nutritional requirements brought about by various kinds of stress are acknowledged in every professional nutrition text. In some persons, certain of these discrepancies are in fact "born in" and are called inborn metabolic disorders. These nutritional imbalances can show themselves in ways so natural and so ordinary that a composite picture of several small discomforts may be required before we begin to pay attention — and even then we may attribute any problems to pettiness or a poor temper unless clear-cut, definite symptoms appear. Many small signs are ignored for years, many years. Ignored, made light of, or treated with over-the-counter drugs until the point is reached when some final tiny insult to the mechanism catapults you into a serious condition while you wonder how it could have happened.

Disease does cause added stress — and stress can quite suddenly cause disease to become evident. Much research has pointed up the fact that diseases that are latent in a healthy body can be brought to a recognizable form by additional stress of many kinds, such as a sudden serious trauma, the wrong kind of weather, losing a job, or an ongoing stressful lifestyle.

It was while making suggestions to people about needed improvements in their diet that I began to recognize how many things were involved for each individual. The diversity of needs is amazing and intriguing. The list includes

- density of nutrients
- the right preparation of foods
- the right choice of particular foods
- ease of digestion
- ease of preparation
- ease of shopping
- ease of eating
- affordability

The need that it was hardest for me to learn was that foods, even foods that should be very good for you, must be enjoyed if the majority of people are to be expected to continue using them in their diets. No matter how good the intention, and the value of the ingredients, some people just cannot stomach some foods no matter how good they're supposed to be. The purpose of this book is to help you to improve your nutritional health in a way that puts the continuation of that improvement under your control. I decided to put this book together using real food, and providing enough variations in suggested eating strategies to allow you to develop a plan that will fit the many situations having to do with you, your heredity, your environment, and all the other individual and unique conditions that make you the person you are. This book is intended to give you the tools to help yourself become — enjoyably — the best that you can be.

A Note on Repetition

A short note to explain my style. There is a great deal of repetition in the course of the book. This is purposeful. Knowledge and practice are separated by a large gulf. It is one thing to learn an idea, but it takes more than simply learning to put that idea to work — to use it on a regular basis. This principle applies to any skill, including taking care of our bodies.

Programs or classes for teaching any discipline, from arithmetic to zoology, rely on going back over points that have been forgotten or whose use has been misunderstood. It takes repetition and practice to master a new skill. The reason is to imbed the proper practice into the fingers as well as into understanding.

This book is most concerned with helping you acquire some day-to-day methods of investigating, improving, and maintaining your nutritional health. Reasons are given to back up the methods, but the emphasis is on the practice — and that requires going over and over some points until they are firmly understood and easy to carry out on a daily basis.

❧ PART I ❧

The Art of Dieting: A New Look

❧ 1 ❧

You Are Unique

Each of us is unique. We are not created equal. Our nutritional needs may be basically the same, but the day will never come when any one of us can be told exactly how much we personally need of any given nutrient under any of a variety of circumstances, such as when stressed, sick, aging, diseased, disabled, pregnant, menstruating, overworked, overheated, overcooled, or living under nerve-racking, noisy, or very busy circumstances. Those individual needs or levels we must try to find by ourselves, by trial and error.

We must eat to live. This book is intended to make it easier for you to fill your own nutritional needs. If you learn what foods are right for you, in what amounts, under constantly changing conditions, you can enjoy every minute of your eating — and live better as a result.

Any part of your body and its workings, with all its delicate timings and switches and seasonal changes, can break down for lack of the right food. It seems only sensible when you have a disease or injury of any sort, when you have pain of any kind, when you have stress, when you have an emotional crisis to go through, when you have hard work to do, even if that work is only to continue existing, one of the first things that should be attended to is diet, which is the key to building, repairing, and maintaining your body.

Even if your diet is good, there seems always to be room for improvement. There are still many diseases whose origin is unknown. Whether or not the cause of a disease is known, a healthy body suffers disease less frequently and less severely than a body starved of one or another nutrient. If the elements we are short of are not added, we cannot rebuild our bodies or even maintain their health. If your body lets you know it needs something by breaking out; hurting; getting too fat, too flabby, or too thin; feeling numb, overly fatigued, or even alien to you because of depression, remember — you are the boss. Learn *what* to do about moving or feeding your body better, and then *do* it!

 Diet is a level on which you can positively help yourself.

All of the eating strategies described in Part II of this book are designed not only, or even mainly, as weight-control diets but as *programs to help you achieve better nutrition.* Good diet can often bring your clinical measures such as blood pressure and cholesterol to normal levels; improve your appearance and energy level; help you eat well in spite of false teeth; help you to remain regular in your bowel habits; help you to live more comfortably with stress or aging.

If you need to lose weight or gain weight, if you need to build or maintain health, with this book you can learn for yourself which particular foods to eat and how much of each food is needed to keep you, as an individual, in the best possible condition.

Get to Know Your Body Type

Your body type depends to some extent on racial and family heredity. There are three basic body types:

- The endomorph is round and soft.
- The ectomorph is extremely slender.
- The mesomorph is solid and muscular.

Most of us are some combination of these. The round, soft types, for example, have the most difficult time achieving a fashionable slender look, but in almost every case that more solid, slender look can be achieved.

Doing It with Mirrors

If you want to get yourself into a better set of habits and better condition, your personal awareness of your habits and your appearance is needed on a continuing basis. Your judgment cannot be accurate without the use of a couple of mirrors, one of which must be at least half your height. A mirror three feet tall will allow anyone six feet or shorter to see themselves from head to toe if it is hung at the right height; a four-foot mirror gives you a little latitude for viewing yourself as you walk toward the mirror, turn, stand tall, wear heels, or exercise. The second mirror can be hand-held, so that you can see the back of yourself from head to heels.

Use Your Own Judgment

The best way to judge your body type, the amount of extra weight you carry, and your condition is to see for yourself. And you can tell — it shows. In the morning, before gravity pulls everything downward, take a good, long look at yourself in a full-length mirror — no clothes! Are you overweight? Underweight? Are your muscles hanging slack from lack of use? You can live a long life and not even be aware of some physical problems unless you see your whole body at one time. It is important to continue to use the mirror almost daily to remind yourself visually of the problems. Some part of you may be weakening or sagging without your being conscious of it. Your muscle tone may be slowly slackening, body fat slowly gathering over little-used muscles, and all you notice without a mirror is that your clothing size is changing.

The extra weight, the slackness of muscle, which you could easily see with a mirror, may be dragging you down, but you may not be directly aware of them. You may just feel a lack of ease in moving, a slowing down, a steadily growing discomfort. Mostly we blame these changes on aging. But they come about almost entirely through a lack of practice in moving, through letting our nutritional condition worsen by ignoring good habits of eating. A mirror is a useful tool. You will tend not to ignore problems that you choose to look at as a daily reminder.

We can't change our inherited body types, but with information about how and why things happen to bodies, and with mirrors to let us see the truth, we can all learn how to adopt the right habits for our own specific set of problems. We can all achieve a measure of success that we may never have believed possible.

Do You Really Need to Lose Weight?

Over many years, in the many people that I have seen, I have never found excess weight of any sort, or a sloppy body, to be the determining factor in love, friendship, or marriage. That does not prevent thousands of us who are psychologically bombarded by constant advertising from thinking that we are ruining our lives by not looking like someone other than ourselves.

Let's stop letting other people lay guilt trips on us. It's true that the insurance statistics tell us that we'll live a little longer, maybe even a lot longer, if we keep our weight low. But there has to be room for variety in life, and most important, there must be room for quality of life.

If you have to be on an unsatisfying weight-loss diet that deprives you totally of your favorite foods, life is not going to be very enjoyable (unless you learn to enjoy deprivation).

If you enjoy the feeling of your thighs rubbing together as you walk, that is your business and your prerogative. If you like the feeling of filling a chair, if you like the warmth and comfort of your body when it is well filled out, *and your health is good,* stay whatever weight feels right for you. It is the right of each of us to choose for ourselves how we will live, as long as we do not ruin our health and so force others to take responsibility for us because we cannot move or have made ourselves sick.

Finding Your Personal Formula
Eating should be a pleasure. Few people want to be concerned about how much food they eat. Savoring the smells of cooking, the sight of food, the different tastes, the feel of food, its texture,

consistency, weight, temperature in the hands and mouth — and providing food to others — these are among life's most enjoyable times, and they supply us with endless memories. Food has always been used as a central theme of family gatherings; weddings, funerals, picnics, holiday dinners, breakfasts in bed, goodies as the solace for the hurts of life. Food is a part of the high points and low points of living and a source of endless conversation as we tell endless pitiful, horrifying, or comic tales about rotten foods we've eaten or times we've had to go without.

For most of us, food is the single most important thread that ties our lives together. It is woven in and around everything we do. *We love food!* And the majority of the people feel guilty about it! Why? Because some of the wrong foods for us as individuals and as groups make us fat, sick, diseased, or depressed. All very good reasons to worry about what we are eating.

We *can* eat, and eat a lot, without getting fat, diseased, sick, or depressed. It takes getting to know your body on a very personal level. It means giving your body all the foods it needs and some of the foods it wants. Is there really such a formula for you?

> • **Calories aren't the only thing that counts.**
> • **What is good nutrition for someone else can get you into trouble.**
> • **Inherited nutritional needs play a large part in determining which diet will fit you.**

That is what we are going to help you find, a way for you that will allow you to eat as much as you wish and yet stay the right weight, build your health, and stay satisfied, happy, and relaxed. Eating should always remain one of life's greatest pleasures!

Don't Blame Yourself

If a diet makes you fat or ravenous, it is not your fault. It is simply a matter of the diet's not being the right one for you. There are people I have met who have tried to exist on 400 and 500 calories a day and yet have become grossly bloated and overweight. One woman was trying her best to lose weight living on 400 calories a day, but in the form of saltines and bouillon. She was carrying pounds of fluids around with her, pounds that came off rapidly once she began eating the right foods, even with five times the calories!

On the other hand, I have met nearly a dozen people who on 4000 calories a day looked scrawny, agitated, and insomniac. They were most often well-intentioned people trying to become vegetarians whose heredity would not allow for the extremes of diet to which they subjected themselves. There are many people who do lose weight on diets and who seem to be doing okay — until they lose their regularity, their hair, and their health. There really is no alternative: you must find the right diet for you!

No one diet is good for everyone. Invariably people living in the same households, in the same families, will have astonishingly different needs. This book tries to provide you with the means to achieve the best possible diet for yourself on a continuing basis.

Starting Off on the Right Foot

Let's assume that you're determined to modify bad habits, heed your body's nutritional needs, and put yourself on the path to better health and a brighter attitude. Good for you! Any journey presents obstacles, and if you've tried dieting before, you know that an attempt to change your relationship to food poses more problems and temptations than nearly any other quest. Here are a few suggestions to help you along the way.

Be Proud of What You Do for Yourself
You are unlikely to stick to any habit, no matter how good, if you constantly feel sorry for yourself or if the habit is distasteful to you. If, for instance, you're going to lose weight successfully and keep it off, you can't hate what you're doing or pity yourself, or have other people pity you. If you want good habits, you must take pride daily in each of your small successes.

You don't want to go for instant satisfaction and continue out of control in your eating habits, but also you should not opt for constant, long-term misery, feeling that you must suffer if you are going to have good eating habits. Either way, you become a burden to yourself and to everyone around you. Who needs it? You don't, and neither do the people who care about you.

There is great satisfaction in treating yourself intelligently, feeling better and happier and healthier, day by day and year by year, and knowing that you have done it all for yourself!

RECOGNIZE THE EXCUSES

Never, ever again say . . .

I'll buy this just for the guests.
I'll fix a snack for the kids.
I'll have just one.
I can't throw this away.
I can't serve a meal with no dessert.
I've already ruined my diet for today.
I'll just have a small piece.
It'll weaken me if I don't eat.
I have to cook this way for the family.
It costs more money for diet food.
I'll get in shape after I lose weight.
I'll sit for a while before I take a walk.
I haven't got the time.
I have a large frame.
I do sedentary work.
It runs in the family.
I'm too busy.
They like me better this way.
Tomorrow I'll do better.

None of us wants to live having to reject temptation forever. If the wrong foods are in your home, you will almost certainly be tempted daily. Very few people can resist daily temptation. Help yourself to win the health and weight battle by buying for your home only those foods that will build and maintain health. *Keep the wrong foods for you out of your home!*

"I'm Hungry!"

And the call of the stomach is heard throughout the land.... Have you ever tried reading the signals that your stomach sends you?

Shopping Problems. When you go shopping and happen to see a new dessert, some new food that looks interesting, some old favorite you haven't eaten for a while, or maybe a bar of chocolate — you may have just eaten, even stuffed yourself, but your mouth begins to water, you *want* it! That's appetite! You are not *hungry.* You do not *need* food. You *lust* for food! Those moments call for you to exert tight control till you have retrained yourself.

On the other hand, if you have not just eaten, the combination of hunger *and* appetite can lead you to wreck your diet and your budget. You tend to buy more food, and more of the wrong foods, if you shop when you're hungry. This in turn means more food and more of the wrong foods in your home, under your nose, till you or someone else eats them. You don't need the temptation, the frustration! Gain more control over your dieting and your budget. *Eat before you go to food shop.*

"My Stomach Needs Something!" When you're having an argument, when someone has made you unhappy, when you're about to do something exciting, when you're bored — again your stomach may send signals. But stomach signals are not always hunger signals.

When you are in trouble of any sort, your body wants either to fight or run away. These are very natural reactions. As we have become "civilized," instead of popping people in the teeth when they deserve it, or just turning our backs on them and running, we remain polite, try to be understanding, apologize for breathing . . . and many of us eat, and eat, and eat.

You should pay close and intelligent attention to the signals from your stomach. Pain or other responses from your stomach because of anger, fright, unhappiness, injuries, or stress from your work, family, friends, co-workers, or enemies should be considered carefully. If your stomach is not hungry, don't feed it.

If you need to confront someone or some situation, do something about it! It is better to act immediately or to choose a physical response such as a long walk, wild dancing, or singing at the top of your lungs to work off your reaction. *Do not eat when you're upset. It doesn't help you — it will hurt you.*

"Well, I Feel Hungry!" If you have trained your stomach to very regular mealtimes, it will remember mealtimes even when you don't. Let a mealtime come and go without eating because you're busy, and suddenly you notice this terribly empty feeling in your stomach. That is conditioned hunger. "I must be hungry because the time is twelve noon! Feed me!"

"I Am Truly and Honestly Hungry!" If you do not have scheduled mealtimes, you may find that only when you have gone for a period of time without food will your stomach "sit up and beg." That is honest hunger. Your body has run out of raw materials and needs more to keep your systems working.

Don't Fight Distress with Food
From the time we are infants, we are taught to respond to both hunger and distress with food. If an infant cries for any reason, we tend to feed it. This is our way of showing love, of showing concern, of taking care. But should distress, boredom, or anger be dealt with this way? It has been suggested that this may build a habit that will lead to an adult life in which all anxieties and frustrations are met by eating.

It seems that relieving our distress, or if that is not possible, distracting ourselves from distress, with something other than food would be a better way for us to deal with it.

Physical activity helps a lot. Contact sports, in particular, help many people; but a long walk or dancing is great, even at home for those who tend to spend more time alone or secluded. Walks are almost always better when taken with a friend. Many magazine and journal articles lately have pointed out the relaxation of stress brought about by owning an animal that you can pet and take for walks. Human or animal, friendships help a lot.

Coping with Restaurants
You'll need to learn to cope with built-in environmental factors: kids and their school lunches ... workers and cafeterias ...

friends' dinner parties . . . business lunches and dinners . . . after-work cocktails. These are all difficult to deal with until you steel yourself and finally change your eating habits for good.

The worst problems for most people come with restaurant eating. Statistics say that we are eating more than half our meals outside the home. If this is true, we can no longer allow ourselves to be intimidated by waiters, waitresses, or even our favorite restaurants. It is up to us to let them know how we want them to change to accommodate us and our needs. Many restaurants have already changed drastically. We can now find many salad bars where twenty years ago there were none. Even some fast-food restaurants are changing for the better.

When eating out we tend to dream up lots of excuses for continuing to eat food we know we shouldn't eat: "I don't want to bother the waiter," "They probably won't give me something else in place of this," "Well, I've paid for it, I might as well eat it." Yes, you *have* paid for it. So why not insist on getting what you want? You wouldn't let a clerk make you take a dress or a tie that you didn't want, and you certainly wouldn't pay for it and then leave it lying on the counter. Don't pay for food you know you shouldn't eat, and don't eat it just because they serve it. Rather than letting it sit on the table send it back with a polite word: "Sorry, too much salt," "Sorry, but this was overcooked," "Sorry, I didn't want the sauce added."

It is good for your future meals and the restaurant's future business if you let the owner or manager know that other restaurants *are* willing to satisfy your wishes. Let them know how many restaurants are giving a choice of whole-grain breads and crackers as well as refined-flour breads for those who want them. Let them know where you can get varied salads, or where the salad or vegetable appetizers are served first, either in place of or in addition to breads and rolls. Let them know that there are places where sauces and salad dressings are fresh, and most important, served separately, so that you can decide how much, if any, you want to use. Let them know, because your continued business is their continued business.

I make it a habit to discuss with the owners of my favorite restaurants what I admire most about their restaurant and their service and what I consider is hurting them (and, of course, me).

A good restaurateur, even in an inexpensive restaurant, always cares. Yes, there was a time when I wouldn't have dared to make such suggestions! Now I wouldn't consider *not* making them!

The next time you eat at a restaurant, try these techniques:

If there are white rolls and butter on the table when you sit down, pick them up before the headperson disappears and say, "Will you take these with you, please?" It's so much easier than sitting there fighting temptation and your hunger as you wait, first for the menus and then for the food. And in just one virtuous moment you will have saved yourself — how much? Let's say one roll is 80 to 100 calories, one pat of butter is 50 calories. You will have saved yourself 130 to 150 calories.

In just about every restaurant you can order a double salad instead of potatoes, which are usually fried or smothered with cheese, butter, or sour cream. Insist on the salad being absolutely fresh—no brown edges, no wilted edges. A whole salad bowl of greens with a teaspoon of dressing will give you four to five times the nutrients (probably more) than one roll with butter for the same calories.

If you want to avoid some problems, don't order dishes with fancy sauces unless you know that they are low in calories, fat, sugar, and salt. Most sauces (and most salad dressings) can add several hundred calories to an otherwise reasonably low-calorie dish. You can have 75 calories of greens and other vegetables but 200 to 300 calories in a few tablespoons of dressing. It is an easy mistake to make, and most people serving themselves at salad bars do make it. Here are a few suggestions that might help:

- Measure carefully the amount of dressing you use. One teaspoon is enough if you mix the salad well to get dressing on every leaf.
- Choose the thinnest salad dressing you can find, or try oil and vinegar.
- Choose the *fresh* foods — vegetables and fruits — not noodles.
- Don't choose foods that already have mayonnaise or other dressings added for you.

How Do You Refuse Food Offered at Holidays and Celebrations?

Holiday, celebration, and Sunday dinners have changed less over the years than other meals. Everyone has a hard time avoiding overeating at holidays. It is difficult not to get into the spirit of things and join in the feasting. Festival food, especially homemade food, which has taken time and effort to prepare and is meant to bring back old memories, is a love offering. How do you turn down such a gift? A rejection of food offerings is somehow taken as a rejection of the whole: the people, the place, the past, the present, the future.

Call ahead. Appeal to family and friends as far ahead of time as possible. Tell them you're on a special diet and tell them what you *can* eat. Offer to bring it with you. They are trying to please you or they wouldn't have invited you in the first place. Calling ahead takes the blame off you. You are not rejecting their best, most loving efforts. They now know what you can eat. Most people with this information will go out of their way to prepare foods properly for you. If you can't reach them, it may be best to take a gift of foods that you can eat without problems and hope a few other people do the same. Don't let anyone turn your diet into table conversation. It's a bore for anyone not on your diet and rude to those who may need to lose some weight.

Remember, food is offered as a gift. Don't put your hosts in the position of feeling they have mistreated you — or that they are being mistreated by you.

The Care and Feeding of Friends

There is some terrible thing in most of us that makes us encourage our overweight friends' love of eating. We give them larger portions and offer them foods that will make their eyes light up. "Eat! Eat! Afterwards we'll talk about your heart attack."

The pressures of friendship can become very fattening. How many of us can turn down a rich dessert that a friend has fixed especially to please us? It's hard to say no to a friend for any reason, even though we may want to. How many of us have prepared a rich dessert to please a friend, even when we have known that he or she has a weight problem? Most of us are guilty. Special desserts used to be holiday fare. With food easier to come by nowadays, it is uncommon *not* to be offered a rich dessert. Quite often you will be fed the dessert without even having a meal first. Every day has an occasion — a coffee break, lunch with friends, a drink with friends — an occasion to get fat, all in the name of love and friendship!

If you love someone, you may bring them a gift of candy.
If they're worried, you may take them out for a drink.
If they have a birthday, you may give them a cake.
If they graduate, get promoted, have an anniversary, you throw them a party.
If they die, you bring traditional foods to the home of the bereaved.
And if they love you, can these friends turn you down?

 Does love mean always having to say "I'd love some"?

If you love your friends, can you continue to present them with food that you know is going to make them heavier than they should be? That is likely to make them ill? That may even kill them? If you love them, feed your friends as well as you feed yourself. Maybe you should feed yourself better out of consideration for your friends?

✿ 2 ✿

A Closer Look at What We Eat

Use your will power and better judgment to select and eat
only the foods which are best for you, regardless of the
ridicule or gibes of your friends or acquaintances.
— Dr. Richard T. Field

Although we know many of the nutrients needed to keep us
healthy, professional nutritionists assure us that we have barely
scratched the surface of knowing

- what are *all* the nutrients we need
- in what amounts
- in what specific combinations
- at what particular times of our lives
- under what particular circumstances
- for which individual

We can only arrange our diets with the knowledge we have, but
we should also recognize that there must be nutrients or uses of
nutrients of which we are still unaware, or something in the composition of foods or the ways in which we prepare them that we
as yet do not understand fully. That does not have to stop us from
trying to find a better diet for our own unique bodies.

If your health is not established or sustained by the diet you use
daily, you are damaging yourself. A damaged body has more difficulty maintaining normal weight. Any number of diets can be
arranged to contain a wide variety of foods prepared in different
ways while at the same time providing all the nutrients needed to
keep the average person healthy. Yet one or more of those diets
may have *you* feeling either distinctly below par or on top of the

world. Finding the right foods to maintain or build your health is your responsibility. But it is possible in almost every case if you use some of the simple methods shown in this book.

Food "Nut" — or Food Conservative?

There are many reasons for you to consider being something of a food "nut." First, everyone knows that it is several times more expensive to buy all the parts that make up an automobile than to buy the completely assembled car. This applies also to disassembled foods: the separate parts always cost much more than the whole. For instance, wheat bran, wheat germ, white flour, and vitamin E are all sold separately for probably five to ten times what you would pay for plain ground whole wheat, which contains all of them.

More than that, if we are not completely knowledgeable about what foods are composed of, we may leave out useful parts when we buy a product. For instance, we might buy wheat flour, or bread containing it, unaware that almost everything but calories has been stripped away from the original product, which was *whole* wheat flour. After using it for a time, we might have to buy back the bran to relieve constipation and the vitamin E to relieve stiff joints and other ailments. How much wiser and cheaper to buy whole wheat in the first place for our cereals, pilafs, and breads.

From the time we appeared on the earth, our bodies evolved as we ate other living things. Plants and animals are complex systems. As foods they are so complex that biochemists and nutritionists have, even now, merely begun to explain them. Every year new and important uses for nutrients are discovered in the laboratories. Nobody pretends that biochemical or nutritional knowledge is complete, or even nearly complete, particularly about subtle and rare trace elements in foods.

When a food-processing plant strips down a food for appearance or for convenience, some nutrients are destroyed, while others may still reside in the leftovers, which are taken up by another manufacturer, who processes them for vitamins, minerals, roughage, and so on. (We have no way of knowing what important nutrients may be discarded in the second and even third processings.) The disassembled foods are then marketed to us. Buying each of the separate parts is costly. We pay for processing not only in money but also in consequence of not knowing if we have all the useful parts that were once in the unprocessed whole. I think I'm really being a food conservative when I say I see no reason to pay extra in one form or another for the unnecessary taking apart (with possible loss of nutrients) of the food I choose to eat.

The second reason for being a food nut has to do with additives such as colorings, taste enhancers, flavors, preservatives, and the like. These additives are usually synthetic, that is, they are compounds made by manufacturers and not ordinarily occurring naturally. For example, there is a compound that smells like fresh-baked bread. It is put in the wrapper of bread, which can then sit for days on a market shelf getting stale but still smelling fresh. Such compounds are all usually well tested for obvious short-term toxicity, but some problems can elude such testing. It is very difficult to trace the cause of long-term, remote effects. Our bodies, as connected systems, can spread out the time between an insult and its consequences. For example, a single unusual dose of hormones at or before birth can influence greatly the form of sexual maturity many years later. So the effect may not become apparent until long after the cause may be gone or seem to be gone. These connections are hard to track down either by experiment or by statistics. Since we are equipped by nature to deal only with natural hazards (our cells actually choose what to allow through their membranes from the material offered), confronting our bodies with unnatural compounds is a risky experiment.

There is no reason not to take medicines when modern practice affirms them to be lifesaving and useful. But there is also no reason to take unnecessary risks when we are not sick — swallowing substances insufficiently studied because some manufacturer, more concerned with profit than public good, finds an advantage in using them.

And then, we are not all constituted alike. Some people are more sensitive to toxic insults than are others. This also occurs with natural foods. For example, there is a hereditary disposition, among Greeks and Italians in particular, to get very sick from eating fava beans. Or some children inherit an inability to handle certain important amino acids (such as in the disease phenylketonuria). But such idiosyncrasies are hard to discover with respect to unusual manufactured compounds given in low doses. The effect of certain food dyes on the mental state of a few children seems undeniable — but it does not show up in the statistics of ordinary general testing for toxicity. So the second reason for being a food nut is again a conservative one, not to take needless risks.

Finally, because these sentiments are growing among people, some manufacturers take advantage by putting out products whose packaging and advertising seem to promise you something that does not appear inside the package. This is especially treacherous, and it works: there is a well-advertised, popular "old-fashioned" lemonade that has no lemon in it.

Although manufacturers are required to list added chemicals on the package, this is of no help, for who among us — chemists included (I've asked them) — knows what those compounds are or what they do? My academic friends tell me that there is no field so endless and yet so unexplored as the study of commonly used toxic substances. I see no reason to accept additives in my foods if I can avoid them.

More and more, it is important to read and to understand labels and to opt for foods that have the least added to them and the least subtracted from them.

"Every time that a natural substance is removed from a food, every time an adulterant is added to a food, the balance in nature is disturbed. . . . The chemical and cellular processes within the body cells cannot react to the passing whim of chemists without disturbance in function. It took thousands of years for the body to adjust itself to changing environmental conditions. When these conditions are suddenly altered by the actions of men, the cells cannot make the adjustment — disease is the result."

— Dr. Edward J. Ryan

Mother Used to Know Best

Women used to arrive at the right sorts of food for their families according to where they lived, shifting within the locally available diet till they found what kept their families healthiest. Some lived at the seashore, where fish and seaweed were readily available; some in the mountains, where small animals, seeds, and fruits were to be found; others in the plains, where crops could be grown and animals grazed under the direct supervision of the family that was to eat them. Women passed on to their daughters their practical knowledge and the empirical rule "If it works, use it."

It's harder to do today.

Choose Your Own Poison

Three decades ago it was common to prescribe DES (diethylstilbestrol) to prevent spontaneous abortion. It took over twenty years to discover that female children born after DES treatment suffered from a marked tendency to early cancer of the cervix and later from behavioral disorders. Now endocrinologists are finding that male and female laboratory animals given a single large dose of a sex hormone as infants show changes in adult behavior.

Do you think it's not important because it's not used anymore? Then ask yourself whether chickens and cattle artificially fattened by very large doses of the same hormones can be eaten with impunity by us or by our children. It ought to be noted that some male farmers who handled some of these hormones when mixing feed developed enlarged breasts. Now the hormones are packaged to protect the farmer. But what about those of us who eat those hormone-treated animals?

Now, consider the carcinogens. Most of us who are older remember the infamous case of "butter yellow," a dye used to make margarine look like butter. It was so carcinogenic that it was forbidden reasonably soon after its use was begun. But other compounds, less clearly cancer-causing, continue to be used because it takes so much longer to test them. The good news? Fortunately, modern methods have speeded up the testing. The bad news? Unfortunately, new compounds are produced faster than they can be tested. Among the more notorious ones are those used in hair dyes for women. Oddly enough, those used in hair dyes for men are relatively harmless. Since cancer takes so long to appear, chemical agents in foods and cosmetics may have a long run before we find out which ones are at fault.

Next, consider direct chronic poisoning and indirect poisoning by combination. One of the most interesting examples of danger-ous combinations is the injunction that forbids persons taking certain tranquilizers from eating cheeses of any sort. The chemical reason is complex, but think about how such a warning must have come about!

Direct toxicities are common enough. In the 1920s a practice for making cheap chocolate was to dope it with powdered hard coal. Oddly enough, powdered coal does taste somewhat like chocolate when properly mixed with cocoa butter, and it looks a deep chocolate brown. The result was a good deal of kidney disease among children until the use was forbidden. Then there was the case of agene used to bleach flour. This compound pro-duced epileptic seizures in dogs, which is how the effect was found. (Imagine the family dog having fits on white bread left-overs!) Nobody ever implicated agene in human epilepsy, but the baking industry, almost overnight, shifted to other, newer bleach-ing agents.

I have used these examples because they are in the literature and are well over and forgotten, so that they don't concern us directly. But the principle that ought to concern us is the importance of being conservative consumers. We should be wary of purchasing popular novelties or processed products made up of promises and unpronounceable synthetics.

Ignorance Can Be Harmful

In today's world, we don't know whether our vegetables and meats, raised on land which is overused and not completely refer-tilized, are defective in minerals that at one time were abundant in them. For example, there are tomatoes from parts of New Jersey in which iron has been reduced to a trace. Or again, some decades ago, part of the Australian interior was green and beautiful land, yet sheep and cattle sickened and died while grazing there. Then it was discovered that there was no cobalt in the soil. Cobalt is needed in extremely small amounts, but that little amount is necessary for the formation of blood. Once the land was seeded with cobalt, raising healthy herds became possible.

Calories Versus Nutrients

A hundred years ago the manual labor needed for bare subsistence took full time for many families. Lots of calories were burned in this constant work. There was no central heating, so people shivered a lot. Also, fevers ran their course and sicknesses lasted longer. People needed to carry some extra fat to see them through. Accordingly, much more food could be eaten to provide calories, 2000–4000 *more* calories a day than we can consume now without serious weight problems. Today's average need is about 1500–2000 calories a day for most woman office workers or housewives and about 2100–2800 calories for average men who do little physical labor.

Our lives today are sedentary; we get much of our heat from fossil calories (coal and oil) instead of burning our own. We buy prepared foods, we have machines to prepare foods at home, or we eat in fast-food restaurants. Trains, cars, and buses cart us back and forth. Elevators and escalators carry us up and down. Television keeps us sitting still, and electric blankets keep us warm in bed. The power company heats the water we use for laundry, bathing, and cleaning.

The most effective way to burn off the excess calories that we may already be carrying around is to be more active. And our most effective way to prevent adding more fat to our bodies is to lower our intake of calories. We'll go into this in greater detail in Part III. For now, I want to draw your attention to this: *You may need many fewer calories, but you still need to be very well nourished. Those calories must contain concentrated food value if you are to maintain your health!*

Manufactured foods, those that are prepared, preserved, canned, or packaged, have a notable disadvantage: they often contain an excess of calories for the nutrients they provide. They are often refined to improve their keeping qualities, and they must be shipped and then stored for long periods of time. These processes can lead to great loss of food value. Also, the most profitable foods for food companies are usually the least nourishing — refined starches and sugars, with lots of calories and little else but flavor.

If nutrition were a closed and complete science, there would be no need for further nutritional research, an area of study which is growing rapidly. Let us take the nutritionists at their own word, which is that their knowledge is far from complete, and not restrict our diets by using refined foods, for future lists of nutritional necessities will certainly contain many new details.

Some Things You Should Know About Nutrients

Weight loss should never be the only criterion in dieting. It is not good or necessary to lose your health as you lose weight.

The Recommended Dietary Allowances
The book known as *Recommended Dietary Allowances* was first published by our government in 1943 and is regularly revised to give us the best current understanding of human needs for all known food elements. The Recommended Dietary Allowances (RDA) are the *average* daily amounts of certain nutrients that *healthy persons* should eat. This book also presents what it terms Estimated Safe and Adequate Dietary Intakes (ESAD) and other recommendations for some nutrients thought to be necessary for human health. All these suggestions are not *exact* requirements for specific individuals, because such facts are not known. Food needs differ among individuals, and in the *same* individual depending on state of health, age, activity level, and environment. We note, for instance, that as people age, they must be particularly careful to take in enough nutrients, because they need less food to meet lower energy requirements.

Experts are not unanimous about what dietary allowances

should be, and of course their state of knowledge is not complete. We must therefore exercise judgment to supplement available scientific knowledge. Nevertheless, the RDA represent the best available estimate of what human populations must eat to stay healthy, so the diets we offer for your consideration in Part II are all based on the Recommended Dietary Allowances. (Turn to page 291 for some of the RDA nutrient recommendations.)

A good diet for you should not only meet the RDA; it should also give you enough variety in food choices so that you can pick and choose till you have the best selection possible for your enjoyment. Who stays on a diet that they don't enjoy? It is clear that no one eating strategy is right for everyone. Some people sicken on high-protein diets, some on extreme vegetarian diets. Groups of foods, such as vegetables, may be generally good for everyone. Yet you may dislike a particular food in that same group, such as okra, so intensely you won't even try it, or it may make you quite ill even if you love it. *You* are in the best position to choose which foods are best for you. But at least start off with a diet that, like the ones presented in this book, makes good nutrition the priority.

Eat Small, Eat Often

Under the best of circumstances, you absorb only a certain fraction of the nutrients you take in when you eat or drink. The rest passes out through defecation, urination, and perspiration. A good part of the vitamins, minerals, and other nutrients in your food are lost in this way every day. Yet you have some systems that work on a basis of gradual and steady assimilation. Calcium, for instance, after you take it in the form of food or drink, is either stored by your system or excreted within three to five hours. If regular meals are not supplying calcium, it will be pulled out of the storage depots in the bones and other tissues until another meal containing calcium is consumed. Taking all the calcium you need for the day in a single meal or in a supplement once a day will not give you your day's supply. This is why it is important to have three or four meals a day, in order to supply a steady flow of nutrients for those systems that work on the basis of gradual assimilation.

For faster recovery from illnesses, it has long been recognized that the more ill the person, in most cases, the more often that person should eat. Large or rich meals at such a time are seldom tolerated, so common sense dictates small amounts of simple foods served often. It is a simple way to speed recovery. Why not eat this way to build or to maintain excellent health in yourself?

Starve All Day and Get Fat

We hear a big storm is coming that may prevent food from being shipped in. Many of us just can't help ourselves — we start hoarding. We rush to the stores and we grab and hang on to every possible size, shape, and variety of whatever might be in short supply, whether we need it or not, and we store it in our pantries.

Strange to say, your body does more or less the same thing. In fact, almost all living tissues act this way, adapting to existing conditions. When you eat only one meal a day, after the first or second day your body ("What is this person trying to do to me?") becomes very efficient at storing food and less efficient at burning calories. Some food gets used for the daily necessities, but as much as possible is stored away so that if you starve your body for hours again, it can bring these supplies out of storage to keep your systems running. This sort of program is proper for a lifeboat, in the middle of a desert, or during a long winter when food is not often or readily available. Your body is designed to keep you alive under extreme, even catastrophic, circumstances. But near restaurants and grocery stores? Going hungry becomes a formula for gaining weight.

On two meals a day you do a little better, but your body is still not getting its raw materials at the needed intervals and so it again puts food away, in bones, in muscles, *in fat cells,* against future emergencies. You still will tend to gain weight but not as fast as on one meal a day.

On three smaller meals a day *maybe* you can hold your own, but not all of us can.

On four slightly smaller meals a day you suddenly begin to come out ahead.

On five meals a day — five *small* meals — life may become a lot simpler. You feel more satisfied, your stomach doesn't growl the blues, and you may feel better and better. A full stomach does a lot for your moods!

On six small meals a day, using the same number of calories as the one enormous meal that was making you fat, you may never feel real hunger again and your weight will probably come down.

When you eat too much food, some of it gets stored as fat. Strangely, eating too little can have a similar effect. When you eat just enough food, all the nutrients are used up within a short period of time. Little or no fat may be stored. Once food is stored as fat, it becomes much more difficult to get it out of storage.

Eat or Be Eaten

Many systems of the body must have an almost constant supply of a variety of nutrients, for example, the brain, the nerves, the circulatory system. These systems are taken care of without a problem when you are eating the right nutrients on a regular basis.

When meals are missed, or when the right nutrients are not eaten or drunk at regular intervals, your body responds by eating portions of itself! The reserves in your body, stored in your muscles and bone, will first fill the needs of systems that cannot wait. If you miss getting enough of some immediately needed nutrient in your food in one meal, the next meal then should supply enough of the nutrient for the immediate needs of the systems and also try to replace what the body has used up from storage. If only so much of a given nutrient can be absorbed at a time, and you are not eating regular meals, how are you going to catch up?

When systems are not given the opportunity to catch up on necessary nutrients, some damage or weakening will occur, as when bone is weakened by calcium being pulled out for use elsewhere. The accumulation of these damages may finally show itself in a dramatic way, for instance, in the collapsing of a vertebra when a regular loss of calcium has resulted in bones so weakened they cannot support your body weight. For such a thing to happen, the loss must have been going on over a long period of time, but it went unnoticed because there was no pain, no discomfort. Note that the problem will not be confined to just that one vertebra; all the accumulated weakening of all the other bones is still there to be dealt with. A nutrient deficiency attacks the entire body, though it may show itself symptomatically (with pain or other symptoms) in only one or two places at a time.

The weakening and destruction of different parts of the body can happen on *any* diet that does not supply the right nutrients, in needed amounts, at regular intervals. That includes any weight-loss diet that does not take into consideration the body's constant needs. It includes the eating habits many people believe they do well on, such as one meal a day. It includes the meals of people who feel that if it fills you up it's good enough. It includes tea and white toast being used in place of a meal, and those meals of overly refined fast foods that are filled with many calories but few nutrients. For the best health, it is reasonable to assume that you must eat foods rich in particular nutrients and that you must eat fairly often.

Cravings and Binges

It has been suggested that when your body is hungry for substances that you have a special need for, you will tend to binge, but in strange ways that don't fill those needs. Working with people with dietary problems and trying to determine what their needs might be, I have come to feel that this "special needs" theory may be true. If you find that you tend to binge or have strong cravings for particular foods, it may be that you have distorted your *proper* needs with a diet too low in nutrients.

In Part II you will have the opportunity to try several of the diets in this book, all of which are well balanced. If the theory is correct, your need to binge should disappear. For example, if you have been allowing yourself to live on refined carbohydrates, alcohol, sugar, and white flour products, it may take you two to three weeks to get your body back under some control. In this case, the best diet for you to start with will be the Sweet Diet (Chapter 4). It will replace the refined carbohydrates with unrefined carbohydrates and protein, and it should keep you feeling better as your body adjusts to different—and better—kinds of foods.

Go By Your Own Reactions

Milk is an excellent food for some persons, but there are those whose bodies cannot digest milk sugars and those whose cholesterol levels are too high. Where is the justification for making a blanket recommendation that milk is the best way to get calcium when a large proportion of the world's population would be made ill by it? Individual sensitivities and reactions are not to be treated lightly. If only a single woman reports that her child is made somewhat crazy by "harmless" dyes in candy, the answer should not be a diatribe based on the hundreds of children who had no such reaction *that could be observed.* The individual reaction must be taken seriously and should make us watch for this reaction in others. When an individual reports that her headaches are improved upon eliminating a certain food from her diet, again the fact should be noted and added to the list of reactions to watch for. These are empirical data, things that have happened that have not yet been fully explained.

Among our individual differences are requirements for certain nutrients — vitamins, minerals, roughage, and the like. One person can need many times more of a certain vitamin than another person. There is no reliable minimum daily requirement, and some of the "acceptable" minimums can be far too low. Government studies show individual differences to be so wide that any average is meaningless. Those of us who take large doses of vitamins on the basis that not enough has been recommended for more than a few of them are aware that some vitamins have a therapeutic action. For example, vitamin E, sometimes in substantial amounts, can be remarkable in reducing the pain and swelling of premenopausal cystic mastitis markedly and steadily. This observation has been made by many women I know, but it has no official sanction because no study is available to explain it. Similarly, calcium and magnesium have a tranquilizing effect; they are known to lower the irritability of nervous tissue; in fact, magnesium sulfate was once used as a calming agent in epilepsy and rabies. Citric acid promotes the absorption of calcium. But then, very large doses, which can be so useful for some, can be harmful for others.

In reality, each of us is unique, needing different amounts of nutrients, even different foods, according to our genetic makeup, our sex, our age, the way we handle stress, our condition, the part of the country we live in, our water, our air, the season of the year, and the time of the day. And the food itself varies according to how it was grown, stored, shipped, washed, prepared, cooked. Everything counts! How do we cope with this?

In the chapters that follow, we are going to show you several high-nutrition diets. We will also offer suggestions to help you define your personal needs and custom-design a diet strategy that will be one *you* can live with — and thrive on!

❦ PART II ❦

Eight Diets

Nature is kind — much more so than we deserve.
After years of wrong living, she will often reward
us richly for changing our habits and our attitude.
Good health habits alone can add years to your life
and pleasure to your years.

— Dr. Parratt

❧ 3 ❧

About the Eight Diets

You design your own diet. You are the only one who can! You know how you feel. You experience the little odds and ends of things that you know are not right with your system. No one but you can feel them. No one but you can tell when those little things are getting worse, getting better, or when they have disappeared altogether. You who have the direct experience are the best person to change them — and you can!

You will find out, for yourself, what

- makes you feel great
- makes you look shiny and alert
- makes you more energetic
- makes you sleep soundly and wake up smiling
- makes your skin look terrific, tight, alive, and smooth
- keeps your bowels regular and trouble-free
- keeps your digestion so smooth you don't notice it

You are the one who can develop, finally, the right food strategy for yourself, from your own experience — the only way anyone can ever do it.

Dieting for What?

There are many reasons for a person to modify his or her eating habits, most of them having little or nothing to do with the cosmetic effect that usually comes to mind when we hear the word "diet."

You may need to lose weight.
You may need to gain weight.
You may need to develop firmer muscle.
You may need to rebuild muscle tissue.
You may need to lose fluids.
You may need greater than normal amounts of some nutrients.
You may need particular foods to take care of regularity.
You may need foods that you can take without chewing, either now or forever.
You may be trying to eat better on a vegetarian diet.
You may find you need more of certain nutrients as you grow older.
You may have to eat for a time out of cans and packages.

All of these needs and more were considered when this book's eight diets were put together. The diets will allow you to experiment with certain nutrient-rich foods to learn your reaction to them. Trying one (or more) of the diets, while adding your own special touches, will help you become more knowledgeable about nutrition. And, most important, each of the diets offers a low-calorie, high-nutrient core around which you can custom-design an eating strategy that will be both healthful and satisfying, whatever your special needs.

A Brief Look at the Diets

The eight diet plans differ dramatically in some ways and in others are quite similar. One of them may offer the approach you need to get started in developing your food strategy.

Many people do not eat well because of an overwhelming desire for sweet foods. The *Sweet Diet* gives you natural, fresh sweets to feed this hunger, but provides them in the form of unrefined carbohydrates so that they are assimilated slowly and keep you feeling satisfied longer. This diet may help you kick the refined sugar habit for good.

The *Regularity Diet* is especially for persons who suffer from constipation. There is no greater relief than being able to forget about your body functions after you have taught your body to take care of itself. With the right food, irregularity becomes a thing of the past and tasty, filling, fresh foods with lots of roughage, bulk, potassium, water, and some oils become a welcome new way of life.

The *Raw Diet* is a great time-saver. Colorful, delicious, and great for your teeth. If you are a raw food lover, this diet gives you everything you need beautifully. But the diet is not for everyone. You must have access to the freshest seafood and produce; and persons with digestive sensitivities would do best to bypass the Raw Diet.

The *Shine (Anti-Stress) Diet* was designed to help you do just that — shine! For people under stress, people who have been ill or who have chronic debilitating diseases or conditions, this diet may help you to reverse downward trends, or at the very least hold your own. My personal favorite. If you are ill and think a diet like this might help you, please *consult your physician first,* since radical changes in your diet could actually worsen *your particular* condition. You should also check with your doctor to make sure that the high cholesterol content of this diet (many of the most nutrient-dense foods are, alas, also cholesterol-rich) will not be a problem for you.

The *Two-Minute Diet* is easy in every way. It completely gets around problems that sometimes come with aging. There is no cutting or chopping, no chewing, and the liquefied food is very easy to digest. Easy to fix in place of a cup of tea or coffee, this diet takes minutes to prepare and minutes to consume, and is high in nutrients. It is excellent if you are in a hurry. But unless you are unable to be well nourished in any other way, an all-liquid diet should be a temporary expedient at best.

Most men like a diet with the accent on protein. Many versions of high-protein, high-fat diets have been popular for years, even though they are in most cases nutritionally unbalanced. (This kind of diet is actually a popularized version of what was once eaten in the Arctic Circle.) Although I do not recommend such a diet, I am aware that some people will want to try one no matter what I say, so I have included here what I believe to be a better-balanced and more nourishing version than most. The *High-Protein, Low-Carbohydrate Diet* offers more roughage and a better mineral package than most diets of this type. And by using mostly fish (as is used in the Arctic) instead of red meats you can cut saturated fats and cholesterol to acceptable levels. This is not a healthful diet for women, and even in this relatively better-balanced variation I feel it should not be used by men for more than about ten days a year.

The *Pocket Diet* is strictly an emergency diet, based on foods that are highly nutritious though out of cans and packages. It is for people without the time or inclination to prepare simpler foods from scratch. Nutritionally speaking, it is a better diet than many schools and institutions provide and certainly a lot better balanced and cheaper. This is a good short-term answer to life on the run and is an excellent selection for an emergency food storage plan, needing neither water nor a heat source.

The *Lean, Clean Machine Diet* is a great clean-up diet. You will feel satisfied and relaxed on this simple diet meant to supply you with a total range of nutrients at a very low number of calories. In fact, it is too low in calories to be used alone for any length of time, an attribute that makes it excellent as a supplement to your present diet or to any of the others outlined here.

As you can see, each of the basic diet plans has certain strengths and certain drawbacks. Which diet — or even which aspects of a diet — might become part of your life depends greatly upon you, your goals, your needs, your likes and dislikes. Study the diet plans closely, introduce changes gradually, and keep careful records (I'll be giving you suggestions about how to do this).

Good nutrition is the foundation stone of good health. But remember that many illnesses or chronic problems are totally unrelated to diet. Your personal physician or nutritionist should be consulted before you embark on any eating plan that differs significantly from your usual diet.

Trying the Diets

So, how do you get started? I suggest you begin by trying the first diet — or whichever one appeals to you or seems most suitable for your particular problems or idiosyncrasies.

Keep a clear account, a daily record of how you are feeling. Chapter 12 outlines a specific technique for doing this, one I highly recommend. In addition, you will find daily reaction sheets at the end of each diet program. Add questions and other information to the record if necessary. *Don't* rely on your memory — a written record is crucial!

At the end of ten days, try a second diet, again keeping the written records. When you have completed the ten-day cycle on the second diet, compare the two records that you have. You can usually see clearly whether you are better or worse off on one diet rather than on another. The differences as you try out one or another of the diets are sometimes very clear, dramatic, and surprising. One diet — or several — may make you feel terrific. Or you may find that only one or two really work for you.

One or more of these diets, though meeting *known* nutritional requirements, may be lacking in some unknown ingredient that your particular body must have for comfort, and it may not work for you. The variety in the diets and the additional food lists in the final chapter of the book give you the possibility of finding the special food elements your body must have, for that unique balance that will keep you feeling your best. *A daily written record will bring out this important information!*

The Balance of Nutrients for You

The balance of nutrients is about equally good in each of the diets, so far as the known nutrients are concerned. So each separate diet should keep you equally healthy. On the other hand, newly acknowledged food components of great importance are found every year. For this reason the diets use a wide variety of foods.

We all know people who eat the same food as we do, but on those same foods they stay healthy or get sick, get fat or get thin. In other words, we all respond in our own way to different foods, or the same foods prepared differently. Because every one of the diets in this book is high in the RDA nutrients, they are close to equally good in results.

You need not worry about shifting from one diet to another as they are laid out in this book. In our society, at this time, most of us eat out for at least one meal a day, and ethnic restaurants are very common, so changes in diet are not unusual for us. But for all our varied eating, it is important to realize that some of us may

---

IMPORTANT NOTE

There are no two people alike, so if by chance any single food in any of the following diets disagrees with you for any reason, discontinue that food if you know which one it is, and substitute a food from a similar group from one of the many lists in Chapter 17. Shift to another diet entirely if you cannot decide which food is at fault.

The diets are not lifetime prescriptions but tools to help you design a way of eating that will help you look and feel your best.

There are a wealth of options available to you in this book and many alternatives to try.

---

not meet the Recommended Dietary Allowances. Several different studies have found us low in vitamin A, low in folate, low in iron for women, low in potassium, calcium, and magnesium in aging, and low in zinc for older men.

The information in this book is meant to make it simple for you to find the balance you need.

Some Basic Assumptions
Assume throughout all the diets that we mean you to use

- as many fresh vegetables as possible
- fish and shellfish from saltwater sources only
- fresh fruits
- whole grains and legumes
- nuts and seeds, unroasted, unsalted
- skinless young chicken, turkey, guinea fowl
- the leanest meats
- skim-milk, mostly cultured dairy products, including cheeses
- soups and broths only after fat is skimmed
- no standard oil-based mayonnaise or salad dressing
- no deep frying for anything

Getting the Fat Out

Many government agencies both here and abroad are reasonably certain that our high incidence of coronary artery disease, high blood pressure, and stroke is due to the fact that 38 to 40 percent (and I have found among my clients 50 percent) of the calories in our diet come from fat. Think about that! If you eat 1500 calories a day, as many as 750 of those calories are most likely coming from fat! Some government officials cynically believe that we have no hope of changing our diets drastically enough to make much of a difference. They do not believe that we can bring our level of fat intake down to a more reasonable 20 to 30 percent, let alone to 10 to 20 percent. I personally do not just believe but have no doubt that we will bring it down.

When the first studies came out linking fat consumption and blood cholesterol, we Americans started eating leaner meat, or no red meat at all, shifting instead to fish and chicken so enthusiastically we put the entire cattle market at risk. We started going to salad bars, and to fitness centers, giving birth to a whole new, health-oriented lifestyle. And at least partly because of that, our heart disease rate went down!

Our change in buying habits began to change the face of the marketplace. When we stopped buying what we didn't want, better choices became available. Mineral water, unsalted vegetable juices, real fruit popsicles, lowfat dairy products — milk, cottage cheese, yogurt, even cheeses. Everybody got into the act, and heart disease, high blood pressure, and stroke went down still further.

In terms of nutrition, we are a more educated public than we have ever been. We are faced every day with nutritional information coming from magazines, newspapers, radio, television. There are many steps we can take to improve our eating habits. Getting the animal fat out is a giant step in the right direction.

On Which Diet Will I Lose the Most Weight?

Almost invariably, when you are trying several diets in a row, the diet to create the greatest weight loss will be the first one you try. This is because you achieve the fastest weight loss at the time that your body is holding the most excess stored water. Your most readily mobilized energy reserves are sugar reserves (glycogen), which are stored in water, three to four parts water to one part sugar. As your sugar reserves are used up, you don't need the water for storage any longer, so your weight can drop dramatically. In addition, in some people, balancing the sodium–potassium system can cause losses of up to five pounds a day in excess fluids. Two to three pounds a day is not the least bit unusual. This is why many people will lose well during the first ten days of the diet. The loss for most then becomes slower as fat reserves are tapped, since fat is stored in a much smaller proportion of water. A few extremely overweight people may continue water weight loss for as long as six to eight weeks. Carrying stored fluids around makes most of us feel logy and miserable. This should alert you to the fact that sodium in your diet must be cut to a minimum for an extended period of time, maybe forever. A well-balanced diet of fresh, unprocessed foods gives us all the sodium that is considered necessary to our health.

The Lean, Clean Machine Diet, because it is so low in calories, will almost certainly help you to lose the most weight because its calories are significantly less than the others. It is meant to be used as a fast and then only with your doctor's knowledge. For some as yet unknown reason, a diet that is very low in calories (under 1200 calories daily) encourages your body not only to burn calories more slowly but also to give up protein as well as fat.

If weight loss is one of your priorities, be sure to give careful attention to Part III of this book, which examines increased physical activity as an important adjunct to a reduced-calorie eating plan.

More Than One Reason for Eight Diets

It has been suggested that when you change your diet to include foods you do not ordinarily eat, your body takes some time to accommodate. Your digestive system usually adapts to the most efficient ways to deal with this food so as to nourish you and to save some nutrients (including fat) for possible emergency situations. This adaptation takes time, and the effort of adaptation itself could burn more calories. About the time your body has learned to accommodate to a diet and has become efficient in using it, you shift to another diet as different as possible from the one you have been using and weight loss tends to increase again. We see it happen.

One reason for having the variety of diets which we have in this book is so that you can see if trying out one diet after another, forcing your body to accommodate to some extent, will help you to rid yourself of more weight than you would ordinarily be able to lose on a single diet for the same period of time. (*Don't* try this if you are ill. If you try several of these diets in turn, you will have dieted to lose weight for an extended number of days *and you will have been well nourished the entire time.* You will also have learned a lot about which foods your body and all its systems respond well to. Your body may become even more efficient and accommodate more rapidly than you expect. Even so, you should continue to lose weight, although at a slightly slower rate. In the best case, you will lose weight faster and better.

Savings

As has been mentioned, except in the case of some unusual need for a specific nutrient, the suggested diet plans in every case will provide all the nutrients known to be necessary for good health. Since the diets meet the Recommended Dietary Allowances, concentrated nutrient supplements will be needed only in an unusual case. This alone can save you several hundred dollars a year.

The preparation of food by food companies for the market, the frozen, canned, and otherwise prepared foods, costs you many times more than the food in its original form. The diets in this book are prepared mostly from scratch and will save you money. And for the most part, fresh, locally grown, raw foods are higher in nutrients, which means you get more for your money.

There is one more important way in which you will realize savings. Your increasing health will save you trips to the doctor, and that will also save you money.

Quick and Easy Preparation

Most of the meals in the diets take half an hour or less to prepare. Many take much less time. If, as in the Basic High-Potassium Soup recipe (Chapter 14), they do take longer, you may wish to double or triple the amounts and to store or freeze the extra for some other meals.

If your time is exceedingly short, preparing double amounts of food to allow for one hot and one cold meal from the same dish may be a wise option for you to put into practice — but not if having the extra food on hand will prove too tempting.

As you begin trying some of the diets in turn, try not to mix the foods, such as using food from the first diet when you shift to the second. You want clear information about which particular diet(s) work best for you. In some cases you may find foods that are acceptably movable from one diet to the other — as we in fact recommend with the basic soups and certain vegetables. In the experimental phase, since you want to have the clearest picture possible of what your unique needs are, most other foods prepared for one diet should be consumed within the ten-day period allotted for this diet. If you do prepare amounts beyond those you should consume, either put them into the freezer till your trials of the different diets are completed, or, if you think you might be tempted, give them away before starting the next diet. *Take your weaknesses into consideration. Don't put obstacles in the way of your progress.*

Choosing the Best Raw Materials

The human body is a miraculously beautiful machine, with thousands of systems pushing and pulling, moving and holding, building and taking apart, sensing and acting, pumping and grinding, sucking and blowing, vibrating and contracting, sloughing and swirling, working more or less interconnected in synchrony.

The systems and their synchronization are roughly the same for all humans but can be individually quite different. Just a slight disruption in any one system can upset, sicken, or even kill us; in other cases, it may take many small disruptions before the last little change throws the entire system into a more serious problem. Some people seem to have no illnesses, no diseases, in a long and busy life, and others seem to get sick, become allergic, or suffer diseases almost from the time they are born. Heredity plays a strong role. Aside from heredity, environmental pollutants, stress, the wrong foods, and general poverty are very real enemies in this battle for health and even life.

With enormous good luck and by trying our best, we may live out our days in reasonable comfort, keeping mind and body intact. To some extent we can determine our future health by choosing the best of the raw materials available from which to build, repair, and maintain our body.

Choose the simplest, most complete foods, the cleanest water, the right storage (if any), the right preparation, and a quiet and regular time to eat and to digest your food if at all possible.

To Your Taste and Preference

There are some of us who literally hate spinach or sardines or oysters and others who can't get enough of them. There are those who only like a particular food, say onions, raw, some who can't stand it unless it's cooked, and some who just can't stand it, period! Sometimes it's the preparation that turns you off. Some people (many) like chicken or fish broiled but can't stand it boiled. Some can't stand foods mixed together. There can be many different reasons for these preferences, including allergies.

With a public becoming educated to health issues, there are many people now willing to try foods that they may never have tried before, or that they tried as a child and disliked. Tastes change! Our attitudes change! Many children and adults will dislike a particular food on the first taste, but with time and continued contact some of these same foods come to be favorites.

Every unusual food or food with a bad memory attached is worth one tiny trial taste. But you shouldn't feel, or be, forced to finish a food you find disgusting. On the other hand, many times an excellent preparation will change your attitude toward a food immediately. If nothing is going to change the way you feel about a specific food or foods called for in the diet plans, find a substitute that is nutritionally equal from the many lists at the back of the book.

If you are one among the many who have trouble filling their vegetable requirements because you seldom eat *any* vegetables, you'll want to take advantage of the Basic High-Potassium Soup that I recommend in later pages. You can drink your vegetable nutrients in this simple, nourishing soup.

Remember, it's up to you to choose the foods that you find most delicious to fulfill your nutritional needs!

The Diets in This Book and the RDA

Few of us are as healthy as we feel we should be, and most of us are under stress a good deal of the time. The professionals who make up the National Academy of Sciences recognize that differences of opinion exist on the question of whether the RDA should indicate just enough of a nutrient to keep you healthy or whether a larger amount might give you glowing good health and be a more appropriate action to suggest.

Quite ordinarily and on a daily basis we ingest some nutrients in larger than needed amounts. Refined carbohydrates, for instance; fat, for instance; salt; sugar — all tend to be overdone in our usual daily diets. These nutrients are absolutely necessary to our good health, *but not in such overabundance!* On the other hand, there are other nutrients that are not so abundant in our diet but are also known to be necessary to maintain our health. Taking therapeutic amounts of individual vitamins, minerals, and other nutrients in supplement form is sometimes absolutely necessary for good health, and no one with any knowledge of our wide range of individual needs would argue the point. Nonetheless, when taken as supplements rather than in food, the nutrients are often packaged in excessively large doses and almost invariably are more expensive than those same nutrients when bought in food form. Most important, in food form, all nutrients come accompanied by known and unknown helping nutrients.

All of the diets in the following chapters use foods that are

- high in nutrients
- low in fats
- low in salt
- low in sugars
- low in refined carbohydrates
- low in calories
- filling
- satisfying
- eye appealing (for the most part)

And all of the diets make it easy to meet or exceed the Recommended Dietary Allowances, when part of a total eating strategy designed by you along the lines we suggest.

There are some nutrients that are found in few foods and that the body seems to store, such as zinc. These nutrients may be supplied in the diets every few days rather than on a daily basis. Nutrients such as protein or fiber are supplied on a daily basis, as this is the frequency with which they are needed. Nutrients such as calcium and potassium, which are needed at much closer intervals to keep your body functioning smoothly, are supplied with almost every meal.

Food Sensitivities

Excesses are sometimes built into us as individuals, sometimes forced upon us. For example, if someone is allergic to shellfish proteins, any clam can be an excess; and if someone is missing an enzyme for handling milk sugars, any milk can be too much. But also if someone is prone to high blood pressure, most canned foods and restaurant fare are too much, because in the last century salt has become so generally added to food that it is hard to avoid an excess. Prepared foods are, in general, a great blessing for those of us who are not happy when having to cook. But seeing my husband get groggy with violent headaches after eating ordinary popular soups, I began excluding from my kitchen any foods that contain MSG (monosodium glutamate), which is used as a substitute for intelligent flavoring. It is especially dangerous for very young children, if they are constituted like other mammals, for it attacks certain parts of the brain even in small doses.

Awareness of food allergies and sensitivities is a critical part of designing your overall eating plan.

Allergies to Milk

Large numbers of people in the world are allergic to milk and some are also allergic to all milk products. Such people, when drinking or eating milk and foods containing milk, may have problems with digestion, with stuffiness in the nose, phlegm in the throat, and diarrhea. For that reason, the diets in this book widely recommend cultured milk products.

The growth of friendly bacterial cultures in milk products will

ALLERGIES AND DISLIKES

What foods do you dislike? What foods are you allergic to?

If you take the time to write down and keep a list — right here — and to update the list over the years, you will have an individual food history in black and white that will help you keep your health under your control. Your body chemistry is unique. Your allergies, likes, and dislikes have a lot to do with what is good and bad for you. *Listen to your body!*

Symptoms	*Foods*		
Hurts my teeth:	_____	_____	_____
Makes my throat raw:	_____	_____	_____
Makes me cough:	_____	_____	_____
Gives me a headache:	_____	_____	_____
Gives me a rash, itchy:	_____	_____	_____
Gives me heartburn:	_____	_____	_____
Makes me belch:	_____	_____	_____
Gives me a bellyache:	_____	_____	_____
Constipates me:	_____	_____	_____
Gives me diarrhea:	_____	_____	_____
Gives me gas:	_____	_____	_____
I just don't like these:	_____	_____	_____

Ask yourself questions when you feel better or worse in ways you cannot account for. Is it the food? Maybe something it was cooked with? Maybe the pot it was cooked in? Did I wash possible sprays off?

You can sometimes get over or outgrow allergies. Every year or so, try this: Take just one of these foods in very small amounts. If no bad response occurs, increase amounts gradually every four or five days. Your chemistry may have changed so that this food no longer bothers you.

often render them safe for people who are otherwise allergic. Make sure any pasteurizing is done before the culture is added, otherwise the culture will be killed off by the pasteurization. Do not hesitate to call the dairy and ask. Also be sure the milk products are lowfat or nonfat to cut fats, calories, and cholesterol. Cultured products are a practical way of introducing large numbers of particular organisms into the intestinal tract, and are sometimes used to regenerate the proper balance of the intestinal flora after any condition that upsets the microfloral balance in the gut, particularly the use of antibiotics. Good choices in cultured milk products, which you will see mentioned throughout the diets, include:

buttermilk (comes in lowfat or nonfat variations)
kefir (may not be available in lowfat form — give it time)
laban (thickened yogurt or yogurt spread)
yogurt (lowfat and nonfat varieties available)
sweet acidophilus milk (can taste just like regular milk)

If you are so sensitive that cultured milk products give you problems, leave even those products out of your diet. Try them again after a time; your ability to tolerate them may have changed.

There is another problem with all milk products: they do not have a good calcium–magnesium balance. For that reason, be sure your diet includes at the same time foods high in magnesium. You will find a list of such foods in Chapter 17.

Calcium is, however, a vital nutrient. If you can't (or don't want to) use milk products, a list of high-calcium foods is also in Chapter 17. Another good calcium source is the soups described on page 228. There are many other nutritional elements in these easy-to-drink soups which surprisingly, even when made just from vegetables, can give you as much calcium, or even more, than milk.

Allergies to Wheat and Other Grains
Many people are allergic to wheat products. It is the wheat gluten (wheat protein) that is most often the culprit. Corn, oats, rye, barley, buckwheat, even rice, may also cause problems to a lesser extent. But many persons are not aware of their sensitivity to

wheat and other grains and live a mildly sick or uncomfortable life, never guessing that there really is something not quite right about the state of their health. Living full time with a problem whose cause they are not really aware of, most people will accommodate themselves to feeling slightly ill and will accept it.

I have purposely arranged the diets in this book so that if you have this trouble you can eliminate wheat and its by-products (and other grains, if necessary) from the diet you design for yourself.

If you are at all suspicious about your own tolerance for wheat, try whatever diet you choose first without any wheat products. After this trial period try adding small amounts of wheat and see if there are any observable differences. If you are convinced you have no reactions to wheat, the number of calories in the diets is low enough so that you can safely add two slices of bread per day if you feel a need for it. (A number of other grains are listed in Chapter 14.) There are many alternative (and delicious) grain crackers on the market now, especially in health food stores, which use rice as a base instead of wheat. Watch, though, what you put on them, if you use anything at all. The diets have a very healthy balance of fats and oils. Try not to upset that balance by adding extra butter or margarine.

Trouble for Some with the Cabbage Family

If you are at all hypothyroid, the cabbage family has the tendency to lower thyroid production and slow you down. If you are hypothyroid it might be wise to limit your intake of cabbage, cauliflower, Brussels sprouts, broccoli, and kale, plus rutabaga and turnips.

A Closer Look at the Diets

In the following eight chapters, you will find eight different ten-day diet plans. As mentioned earlier, each of these diets has been developed to offer you a high-nutrient, low-calorie core that you can use to develop the eating strategy that suits you best. Each diet plan consists of several major elements.

Shopping List. The shopping list provides a listing of all the foods called for in the daily meal plans as well as some other foods that would be good additions or substitutions to the diet.

Daily Menus. Complete menus for ten days' meals are given next. Remember, these menus represent the nutritional framework for your eating plan; rounding out each day's meals will be the foods *you* select, based on your tastes, your goals, and your own awareness of your needs.

Nutrient Analysis. Following the menus are tables showing the average amount of nutrients supplied daily by the basic diets without any additional foods you might include, and also the nutrients supplied if you choose to follow my recommendation to supplement the diet with a particularly nutritious soup I've developed. Although the nutritional values in the tables have been carefully calculated and appear to be very exact, remember that the figures can at best be only close approximations. The amount of nutrients actually found in a specific food can vary substantially from the agreed-upon norm (all apples are *not* created equal!), and the food choices you make when the menus give you an option will have some bearing too. Because the averages are derived from the ten-day total for each nutrient, your actual day-to-day nutrient intake will vary somewhat from the given figures. Nonetheless, you can be generally confident that through the course of the ten-day diet you will be getting *at least* the average daily amounts listed.

The tables also show how the nutrients supplied by the diet match up to the RDA for men and women aged 23 to 50 (other persons can find their RDA figures on page 291). By following a few simple recommendations, both men and women will easily fill all their daily requirements.

Customizing the Diet. Guidelines to help you analyze and fulfill your caloric and nutritional needs follow each diet's nutrient analysis.

The diets are meant first and foremost to build and to maintain health. Second, as they are laid out, they are ideal as the basis for a weight-loss diet. With simple adjustments these diets will also work superbly well for weight maintenance and even for a gain in

HOW MANY CALORIES DO YOU NEED?

This chart is meant to give you a general idea of how many calories — the least and the most — you should consume. Obviously, if you are overweight at this time, your intake of calories should be at the lowest end of the range. If you are underweight, your intake might need to be at the higher end of the range or beyond. You are an individual. Your needed rate of caloric intake is unique to you and tends to change with age and physical condition. Change the diets according to your needs, adding or subtracting calories but never letting nutrient level drop too low. (For another way of determining your calorie needs, see Chapter 12.)

Recommended Calorie Intake

Category	Age (years)	Weight (lb.)	Height (in.)	Energy Needs (Range) (calories)
Males	15–18	145	69	2800 (2100–3900)
	19–22	154	70	2900 (2500–3300)
	23–50	154	70	2700 (2300–3100)
	51–75	154	70	2400 (2000–2800)
	76+	154	70	2050 (1650–2450)
Females	15–18	120	64	2100 (1200–3000)
	19–22	120	64	2100 (1700–2500)
	23–50	120	64	2000 (1600–2400)
	51–75	120	64	1800 (1400–2200)
	76+	120	64	1600 (1200–2000)
Pregnancy				+300
Lactation				+500

Source: Adapted from Committee on Dietary Allowances, Food and Nutrition Board, *Recommended Dietary Allowances* (ninth revised edition), Washington, D.C., 1980. Consult that book for full information on how the figures were derived.

weight. The average daily calories provided by each diet core are as follows:

Sweet Diet — 827
Regularity Diet — 504
Raw Diet — 852
Shine (Anti-Stress) Diet — 908
Two-Minute Diet — 1080
High-Protein, Low-Carbohydrate Diet — 1208
Pocket Diet — 988
Lean, Clean Machine Diet — 491

Since in general women should not consume fewer than 1200 calories a day and men no fewer than 1500, except under a doctor's supervision, most people, especially men (even those on a weight-loss program), will need to add calories to the core diets. For an approximation of what your caloric needs might be, see the table on page 50.

To fill any slack in the diet, both men and women are urged to turn first to what I call the Choice Filler Foods: a group of selected high-nutrient vegetables (the High-Potassium Foods on page 226) and a super-nourishing soup (the High-Nutrient Soup, page 228), chosen because of their ability to provide high appetite satisfaction and concentrated nutrition at a low caloric cost. In fact, just half the daily soup recipe added to any of the first seven diets will fill virtually all nutritional needs while adding only 245 calories. (The soup *is* the eighth diet.)

These recommendations as well as others are spelled out with each of the diets. The eight diets were developed particularly for those of you who want a simple way to decide what eating strategy or strategies are best for you. You will probably need the ten-day periods of practice with each diet you try and with the Choice Filler Foods. Take your time! This step is very important.

Take the next step only after you have found which diet or diets are best for you. Search out particular nutrients for which you may have a special need or desire in the lists of foods in Chapter 17 and add them to your preferred diet. If the calories in your diet do not allow the addition of a food you want or need, you can exchange one food for another in your diet. Make sure nutritional content is as equal as possible. I do not believe it proper, necessary, or kind for anyone to ever be forced to go hungry. The Choice Filler Foods you can eat at will. These foods are recommended on a daily basis to fulfill your nutritional needs and to keep you feeling satisfied all day (and, if necessary, all night). With these foods, you can meet your needs for quantity and still remain within the necessary calorie limits.

How Is the Diet Going? Each diet chapter also provides a place for you to keep track of your progress. A daily checklist helps you become more aware of how your body is responding to the diet, which will make it easier for you to compare diets and find what's right for you. You can also track your daily weight change on a chart that is provided. It is slightly unfair to chart ten-day diets, since the effects of a diet can often be delayed until the body accommodates. But it is better to know what is happening than to rely on what you *think* might be happening. So we suggest you use the charts and checklist. They are a rough guide, but they are a guide.

Now, on to the diets!

❧ 4 ❧

The Sweet Diet

Around ten days to two weeks into any diet or any change in eating patterns, most people will find it hard to continue with their improved habits, especially if their new diet is low in carbohydrates, starches, and sugars.

Your body requires a certain amount of sugar to feed your brain. It is said that the minimum amount of carbohydrate needed is about 50 grams daily, but there is the possibility that some individuals may need as much as 100 grams or more. Most of us can live in good health on carbohydrate-high foods if we choose our carbohydrates carefully and keep them at about 50 percent of our daily calories.

Carbohydrate Addiction?

The problem is that *refined carbohydrates*, which are pulled into the system with exceeding rapidity, are also, for a lot of us, seemingly addictive. Cleaning your diet of most refined carbohydrates all at once is like going "cold turkey" with any addiction. You may become pale, shaky, nervous, irritable and have a violent craving for just those foods that you are trying to deny yourself. Some people are much more strongly addicted than others, but anyone will do better on a diet of high-carbohydrate foods that are not refined. Some who are determined, who have the right incentive and enough support, will push through and come out with good control over their carbohydrate intake reasonably quickly. For others the going will be rougher.

☞ | **Work with your body carefully. Fulfill its needs.** | ☜

If carbohydrate addiction is a problem for you, try the Sweet Diet. If that is not the answer, try next the Regularity Diet (Chapter 5). Each is high in different types of unrefined carbohydrates.

If You Have Low Blood Sugar

People with low blood sugar tend to overreact to a rapid intake of sugar into the system, for instance when they eat refined and quickly accessible sugars such as those found in ice cream, candy, and most soft drinks; or in cakes, cookies, and muffins; or when they drink alcoholic beverages.

These individuals, who get a good immediate response to sugar intake but a strong "fly-back" afterward, need sugar that is slowly released to minimize or even avoid the fly-back. Fructose, or fruit sugar, is twice as sweet as the same amount of sucrose (widely used in processed foods) and is so well stored in fruit that it is utilized by the body at a steady slow rate.

The Sweet Diet provides the slow release of sugar necessary to run your carbohydrate-using system without sudden peaks and valleys. The diet purposely calls for plenty of fresh fruits. Dried fruits give you much too fast an access to the sugar, so are not appropriate.

A sweet way to diet!

Shopping List
A bullet (•) indicates the specific foods called for in the daily menus. The other listed foods would be good additions to the core diet.

SEAFOOD (ocean fish only)
fish (all varieties)
shellfish (all varieties)
• clams
• oysters
• shrimp

MEATS (very lean)
lamb
liver

POULTRY (young birds, skin removed)
• chicken
• chicken livers
• guinea fowl
• turkey breast

DAIRY PRODUCTS (all lowfat, no added salt or sugar; cultured if available)
buttermilk
cheeses
• blue or roquefort cheese
• cheddar cheese
• cottage cheese
• ricotta cheese
kefir (a cultured drink)
laban (thickened yogurt)
• milk
sweet acidophilus milk
• yogurt

VEGETABLES
asparagus
bamboo shoots
Brussels sprouts
cauliflower
• celery
chard
chili peppers
Chinese cabbage
collard greens
• cucumbers
endive
• garlic
kale
• kohlrabi
• lettuce, looseleaf
mung sprouts
• mushrooms
mustard greens
• parsley
• peppers, sweet green and red
radishes
• scallions
spinach
• watercress
• zucchini

FRUITS (fresh only)
• apple
• apricots
• banana
• blackberries
• blueberries
• cantaloupe
casaba melon
cherries
figs
• grapefruit
grapes
• mango

• oranges
papaya
• peaches
• pineapple
• plums
• strawberries
tangelos
• tangerines
watermelon

NUTS, SEEDS, AND GRAINS (unroasted, unsalted)
• brown rice
millet
• nuts (all varieties)
oat bran
• seeds (all varieties)
• wheat bran (fine)
• wheat germ (toasted)
• whole-grain crackers (no-fat)

OILS AND FATS (in order of preference)
• olive oil
• peanut oil
• light or dark sesame oil
• butter

OTHER
• apricot nectar (canned, no sugar added)
• blackstrap molasses
• fresh ginger
• fresh rosemary
• tofu (firm)

Daily Menus

The basic recipes and food lists referred to in the menus may be
found in Chapter 14.

Day 1

BREAKFAST

Sprinkle:

   ¼ cup your choice from Nuts and Seeds list

   3 fresh apricots, cut up or mashed

over:

   ½ cup yogurt

LUNCH

Cut up raw vegetables:

   1 rib celery

   ½ zucchini

   ½ cucumber

   ½ sweet green pepper

Toss vegetables with (or dip them in):

   Low- or No-Calorie Salad Dressing

Accompany with:

   ½ cup milk

   ½ banana, sliced

DINNER

Bring to boil in small saucepan:

   ¾ cup water

   ¼ cup apricot nectar

Add and cook, covered, till done (45 minutes):

   2 tablespoons raw brown rice

Stir in:

   1 tablespoon fine wheat bran

Serve with:

   ¼ pound cooked turkey breast

SNACK

Mix together:

   ½ cup yogurt

   ½ cup fresh pineapple chunks

Day 2
BREAKFAST
Mix in blender:
>¾ cup milk
>¼ (or less) cantaloupe

LUNCH:
>⅓ cup cottage cheese
>Fresh fruit (choose between 2 plums, 1 peach, 2 apricots,
>   ¼ cantaloupe, or 3 spears fresh pineapple)

DINNER
Preheat in wok or heavy skillet:
>1 teaspoon dark sesame oil
Add and stir-fry till lightly browned:
>1 clove garlic, thinly sliced
>1-inch piece fresh ginger, peeled and thinly sliced
Toss in and stir-fry briefly:
>¼ cup each, thinly sliced: kohlrabi, celery, zucchini
Then add:
>1 tablespoon crushed pineapple
>¼ pound chicken, in thin slivers
*Continue stir-frying till chicken is done and
   vegetables are crisp-tender, about 2–3 minutes.*

SNACK
Toss together:
>¼ cup firm tofu cut in ½-inch cubes
>2 fresh apricots, cut up or mashed

Day 3
BREAKFAST
>¼ pound fish, poached
>2 slices orange

LUNCH
Mix in blender:
>½ cup milk
>½ cup fresh pineapple chunks

DINNER
Mix in morning and refrigerate:
    ½ cup cottage cheese
    1 ounce blue or roquefort cheese
Serve cheese dip with:
    2 cups (or more) your choice of vegetables
        from the High-Potassium Foods list

SNACK
Mix together:
    ½ cup yogurt
    1 peach, cut up or mashed

Day 4
BREAKFAST
Toss together:
    ¼ cup your choice from Nuts and Seeds list
    ¼ banana, mashed
    ½ cup yogurt

LUNCH
Mix in blender:
    ½ cup milk
    ½ cup strawberries

DINNER
    ¼ pound peeled shrimp, steamed
    ½ cantaloupe, cut in thin slices
    Sprigs of fresh rosemary

SNACK
Mix in morning and refrigerate:
    ½ cup cottage cheese
    ½ cup minced clams, cooked and drained
        (or use canned)
Serve clam dip with:
    Your choice of vegetables from the High-Potassium Foods
        list

Day 5
BREAKFAST
Mix in blender:
>½ cup milk
>1 peeled tangerine *or* ½ thinly peeled orange (don't discard the white substance just under the peel; it's high in bioflavonoids)

LUNCH
Mix together:
>½ cup cottage cheese
>½ banana, mashed

Serve with:
>Cut-up parsley (as much as you want) *or* dark green looseleaf lettuce

DINNER
Cook together gently:
>¼ pound chicken livers
>1 teaspoon oil or butter

Then add:
>3 or 4 slices apple (with skin)

Simmer till done to your liking.

SNACK
Mix lightly:
>¼ cup your choice from Nuts and Seeds list
>¼ cup berries, your choice
>½ cup yogurt

Day 6
BREAKFAST
Stir together:
>½ cup hot milk
>1 tablespoon blackstrap molasses *or* 1 serving from Fresh Fruits list
>¼ cup toasted wheat germ
>¼ cup fine wheat or oat bran

LUNCH
Mix together:
    ½ cup yogurt
    1 serving from Fresh Fruits list, your choice

DINNER
Preheat in wok or heavy skillet:
    1 teaspoon dark sesame oil
Toss in and stir-fry till lightly browned:
    1 clove garlic, thinly sliced
    1-inch piece fresh ginger, peeled and thinly sliced
Add and stir-fry till done to your liking:
    3½–4 ounces firm tofu, cut in ½-inch cubes
    1 cup sliced mushrooms
    2 cups (or more) your choice of vegetables from the
       High-Potassium Foods list, thinly sliced

SNACK
Mix in blender:
    ¾ cup milk
    ½ cup fresh crushed pineapple (freeze the
       pineapple first for a great iced shake)

Day 7

BREAKFAST
    ⅓ cup unsweetened blueberries or blackberries
    ½ cup yogurt

LUNCH
    ⅛ pound cheddar cheese
    1 portion fresh fruit

DINNER
Cook lightly together:
    ¼ cup oysters
    1 teaspoon butter
Then add:
    ¾ cup hot milk

Heat again and serve. Accompany with:
> All the vegetables you want from the High-Potassium Foods list
> Low- or No-Calorie Salad Dressing

SNACK
Hot cereal made by stirring together:
> ¼ cup your choice from Nuts and Seeds list, ground
> ¼–½ cup hot milk
> 1 serving from Fresh Fruits list

Day 8
BREAKFAST
> 1 serving from Fresh Fruits list, cut up
> ½ cup yogurt

LUNCH
> ½ cup cottage or ricotta cheese
> ½ cantaloupe

DINNER
Mix together:
> 2 cups or more Basic High-Potassium Soup, heated
> 1 tablespoon fine wheat bran
> 1 heaping tablespoon mixed grains from Whole Grains list

Accompany with:
> 1 serving from Fresh Fruits list

SNACK
Toss lightly:
> 3½–4 ounces firm tofu, cut in ½-inch cubes
> ½ mango, cut in small pieces

Day 9
BREAKFAST
Combine:
>½ cup hot milk
>
>1 tablespoon fine wheat or oat bran
>
>¼ cup toasted wheat germ

Add:
>1 tablespoon blackstrap molasses *or* 1 serving from Fresh
>   Fruits list

LUNCH
Mix together:
>3½–4 ounces firm tofu, cut in ½-inch cubes
>
>1–2 cups Basic High-Potassium Soup, unstrained

DINNER
Cook together covered, until done (45 minutes), then set aside:
>2 tablespoons raw brown rice
>
>1 tablespoon fine wheat bran
>
>¾ cup Basic High-Potassium Soup, stock only

Preheat in wok or heavy skillet:
>1 teaspoon peanut (or other) oil

Add and brown lightly:
>1 clove garlic, thinly sliced
>
>1 scallion, thinly sliced

Stir in and cook quickly:
>½ sweet red pepper, thinly sliced
>
>½ sweet green pepper, thinly sliced
>
>1 cup Chinese cabbage, shredded

Add:
>¼ pound chicken, cut in shreds or chopped
>
>¼ cup fresh pineapple chunks

Stir-fry till just done. Pour over or mix with reserved rice.

SNACK
>1 serving from Fresh Fruits list

Day 10
BREAKFAST
>¼ pound poached fish
>
>½ grapefruit

LUNCH
>1 whole-grain, no-fat cracker
>
>1 handful watercress *or* as much lettuce as you want
>
>½ cup cottage or ricotta cheese
>
>½ banana

DINNER
Prepare:
>¼ pound fish
>
in any of the following ways:
>>*braise in 1 teaspoon butter or oil*
>>
>>or *poach lightly in Basic High-Potassium Soup broth*
>>
>>or *bake without oil or fat in 200°F oven*

Serve with:
>1½ cups melon salad
>
>Low- or No-Calorie Salad Dressing

SNACK
Fold together:
>½ cup fresh, crushed, partially frozen pineapple
>
>½ cup cottage cheese or yogurt

Nutrient Analysis

These tables show the average daily nutrients supplied by the Sweet Diet so you can see how they compare with standard recommendations. Figures include the nutrients provided by the basic diet as listed in the daily menus, and the nutrients supplied if my recommendation to use the High-Nutrient Soup as a supplement is followed. The averages are based on the ten-day total for each nutrient, and the figures have been rounded off. (For a fuller discussion of what the figures mean, turn to page 49.)

The Sweet Diet:
Meeting Your Needs for Nutrients Having Established RDA *

	RDA		Daily Average Supplied by Diet	
Nutrient	Woman Aged 23–50	Man Aged 23–50	Basic Diet, No Additions	Total with Soup Addition
Vitamin A	4000 IU	5000 IU	7750 IU	17,790 IU
Vitamin B-1	1.0 mg	1.4 mg	0.86 mg	1.4 mg
Vitamin B-2	1.2 mg	1.6 mg	1.33 mg	2.33 mg
Vitamin B-3	13 mg	18 mg	9.9 mg	16.7 mg
Vitamin B-6	2.0 mg	2.2 mg	1.4 mg	2.4 mg
Vitamin B-12	3.0 mcg	3.0 mcg	5 mcg	9.5 mcg
Vitamin C	60 mg	60 mg	214 mg	434 mg
Calcium	800 mg	800 mg	824 mg	1232 mg
Vitamin D†	200 IU	200 IU	—	—
Vitamin E	11.9 IU	14.9 IU	13.4 IU	18.8 IU
Folacin	400 mcg	400 mcg	256 mcg	585 mcg
Iodine†	150 mcg	150 mcg	—	—
Iron	18 mg	10 mg	10.3 mg	18.1 mg
Magnesium	300 mg	350 mg	297 mg	502 mg
Phosphorus	800 mg	800 mg	1120 mg	1495 mg
Protein	44 gm	56 gm	64 gm	79.3 gm
Zinc	15 mg	15 mg	12.2 mg	17.5 mg

　　Nutrient values of daily menus were calculated with Health-Aide nutrition software, Programming Technology Corporation, San Rafael, California, 1982.

　* The Recommended Dietary Allowances (RDA) are taken from Committee on Dietary Allowances, Food and Nutrition Board, *Recommended Dietary Allowances* (ninth revised edition), Washington, D.C. Complete information for age groups other than those listed here, and for pregnant or lactating women, may be found on page 291.

　† Nutrient values for vitamin D and iodine are indeterminate, but it is very unlikely that anyone will get less than the full RDA daily if milk or fish is included in the diet.

gm = gram　　IU = international unit　　mcg = microgram　　mg = milligram

The Sweet Diet: Other Important Nutritional Needs

Nutrient	Recommendation*	Daily Average Supplied by Diet		Comment†
		Basic Diet, No Additions	Total with Soup Addition	
Calories	Varies	827	1072	Add treats or needs or both to bring calories to desired level
Carbohydrates	Approximately 58% total calories	88 gm	138 gm	Carbohydrates = about 51% daily calories
Crude Fiber	6 gm or more	6 gm	12.5 gm	Strain the soup if it has too much roughage for you
Potassium	1875–5625 mg	2764 mg	5085 mg	Stay on the high side
All Fats‡	Not to exceed 30% total calories	28 gm	30.1 gm	
Saturated	Approximately 10% total calories	8 gm	8.1 gm	Fats = 25% daily calories (7% saturated, 7% monounsaturated, 5% polyunsaturated)
Monounsaturated	Approximately 10% total calories	8 gm	8.3 gm	
Polyunsaturated	Approximately 10% total calories	6 gm	6 gm	
Cholesterol	300 mg maximum	160 mg	170 mg	Keep on the low side
Sodium	1100–3300 mg maximum	725 mg	1011 mg	Keep on the low side
Sugar	Not to exceed 10% total calories	4 gm	4 gm	Sugar = 1.5% daily calories

Nutrient values of daily menus were calculated with Health-Aide nutrition software, Programming Technology Corporation, San Rafael, California, 1982.

* Nutrient Recommendations regarding carbohydrates, fats, cholesterol, and sugar are part of the Dietary Goals for the United States, prepared by the Senate Select Committee on Nutrition and Human Needs, 1977. Other recommendations are broad guidelines as reported in *Recommended Dietary Allowances.*

† Percentages are based on total with soup addition.

‡ Because values are not available for some minor fatty acids, the amounts listed in each group do not add up to the total for all fats.

Customizing the Diet

CALCULATING CALORIE NEEDS

1. Enter here your daily calorie needs or goals: _____
   (Use the table on page 50, or follow the guidelines in
   Chapter 12 for finding your personal balance. Remember, for best health results, women should generally consume no fewer than 1200 calories daily, and
   men no fewer than 1500, for any extended period.)
2. This is the average daily number of calories in the
   basic diet, without additions: 827
3. Subtract step 2 from step 1 to learn how many addi-
   tional calories daily you will require, on average: _____

FILLING YOUR NEEDS: SOME SUGGESTIONS

1. As shown in the nutrient analysis tables, adding *half* the High-
   Nutrient Soup recipe (page 228) *daily* completes virtually all
   nutritional requirements while adding just 245 calories. Men
   will need to add a vitamin B-3 source to be on the safe side.
2. If you choose not to use the High-Nutrient Soup, the lists in
   Food Sources of Major Nutrients, Chapter 17, will help you
   select foods to meet your nutritional needs. You could, for
   example, forgo the soup and round out nutrient requirements
   by adding these foods to the daily diet:

   > ½ pound raw kale
   > 1 cup raw asparagus
   > 1 cup raw green beans
   > 1 oyster or other zinc-rich food

   Women should also add iron-rich foods. The oyster and
   green beans listed above provide some iron, which could be
   supplemented daily by 1 cucumber or ½ cup chopped parsley
   or 1 cup raw watercress or spinach.
   Two or three times during the ten days, men should also add
   ¼ pound turkey or tuna or other vitamin B-3 source.
3. Once you are sure your nutrient needs are taken care of, you
   can add other foods you like to bring your calorie intake to the
   desired level. The lists in Chapter 14 will help you make good
   choices. This diet has a good balance between carbohydrates,
   protein, and fat; try to maintain that in the choices you make.

How Is the Diet Going?

The checklists and chart will help you keep track of how you're feeling and how you're doing on this diet. Paying close attention to your body's signals may help you determine whether this is the diet for you.

The Sweet Diet:
Daily Checklist of Negative and Positive Factors

	DAY									
NEGATIVE FACTORS	1	2	3	4	5	6	7	8	9	10
Constipated										
Diarrhea										
Sleepless										
Irritable										
Itchy										
Sneezing										
Hungry										
Headache										
Blackout										
Gas										
Heartburn										
Bloat										
Weakness										
Fatigue										
Nervous										
Anxious										
Tremors										

POSITIVE FACTORS

Bowel movement*										
Sleeping well										
Stomach satisfied										
Alert, clear-headed										
Feel strong										
Lively										

* 1–3 times/day with regular, well-formed stool

The Sweet Diet: Daily Weight Change Chart

The horizontal line through the middle of the chart represents your starting weight (Day 1). Each day, mark a new point to show how your weight is changing (or not) as the diet progresses. Draw a line from point to point to chart your weight change.

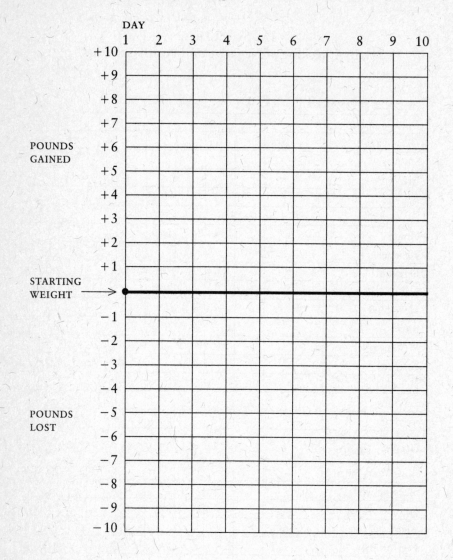

❧ 5 ❧

The Regularity Diet

If there is anything that starts the day off with pleasure, it is the "morning dump," as W. H. Auden put it. Faintly nagging headaches, a bloated belly, and a facial expression of great grimness, coupled with faint anxiety as if an appointment had been missed, characterize the sufferer of constipation. The Regularity Diet, within a few days, gives you bulk and fluid and makes more active the smooth muscle of the gut, all of which help to produce stools that are well formed but easy to pass.

The cellulose and other fiber you find in the complex carbohydrates in this diet may serve as food for animals such as cows and camels but are not accessible to humans as food (at least not yet, though there are many laboratories working on the problem). Humans use these indigestible carbohydrates as bulk and fiber to move the contents of the gut along. The cellulose you get from fruits and vegetables will hold an enormous amount of water. Any unrefined foods of this sort will have much bulk, and bulk pulls in fluids, thereby increasing the size and softness of the stool.

Other animals may have protozoa and bacteria to work on cellulose and related compounds to extract nutrients from them. This does not seem to be the case with humans. We house bacteria mostly in the lower gut, where they make supplemental B vitamins and vitamin K and prevent less useful bacteria from moving in.

After taking antibiotics, which may kill off the bacteria of the lower colon, you should take yogurt to replace the useful bacteria.

A lack of these friendly organisms, which constitute four-fifths of the bulk of the feces, may cause diarrhea and anal spasms.

You need not take the specific food recommendations in the Regularity Diet literally. Many of us have a favorite food that we use to loosen our bowels, such as prunes, figs, bran, scallops, or onions. Surprised? Stranger things than scallops and onions have been used successfully.

Prunes, figs, and bran are traditional because they work for large numbers of people. But no food works for everyone. You may even find that what works for you one day may not work another. Foods that serve only to feed some people will work as a laxative on others, and on still others will literally take the lining off the gut.

In undertaking this diet, it is important to be cautious, especially if your body seems to react strongly to small changes. The Regularity Diet was designed to cover all known contingencies, with a full complement of water, bulk, potassium- and magnesium-high foods, oils, plus a well-balanced nutritional package. Your own personal knowledge of your body will serve to perfect the Regularity Diet for you.

Shopping List

A bullet (•) indicates the specific foods called for in the daily menus. The other listed foods would be good additions to the core diet.

SEAFOOD (ocean fish only)
fish (all varieties)
shellfish
• oysters
• shrimp

MEATS (very lean)
• beef
• lamb
• liver (any kind)
• pork
• veal

POULTRY (young birds, skin removed)
chicken
guinea fowl
turkey

DAIRY PRODUCTS (all lowfat, no added salt or sugar; cultured if available)
buttermilk
cheeses
• blue or roquefort cheese

• cottage cheese
• Parmesan cheese
• ricotta cheese
milk
sweet acidophilus milk

VEGETABLES
• asparagus
• broccoli
• carrots
• cauliflower
• celery
• cucumbers

VEGETABLES (*cont.*)
- garlic
- kale
- kohlrabi
- mushrooms
- onions, red and yellow
- peppers, sweet green and red
- scallions
- spinach
- zucchini

FRUITS
fresh
blackberries
- lemon
raspberries
- strawberries
dried
apples
apricots
figs
pears

LEGUMES
- black beans
kidney beans
- lima beans
navy beans
pinto beans
- soybeans

NUTS, SEEDS, AND GRAINS (unroasted, unsalted)
nuts and seeds
- almonds
Brazil nuts
- caraway seeds
cashews
pecans
pumpkin seeds
sesame seeds
sunflower seeds
grains
- barley
- brown rice
- corn grits (whole-grain)
- cornmeal (whole-grain)

- millet
- oat bran
- oatmeal
- rice bran (fine to coarse)
- rolled oats
- rye berries
- wheat berries
- wheat bran (fine to coarse)
- wheat germ (toasted)

OILS AND FATS (in order of preference)
- olive oil
- dark sesame oil
- butter

OTHER
blackstrap molasses
- curry powder
- dill
- horseradish
- tofu
- tomato paste

Daily Menus

The basic recipes and food lists referred to in the menus may be found in Chapter 14. A double boiler is ideal for cooking grain cereals; it prevents scorching and helps retain nutrients. A pressure cooker will greatly reduce cooking times for soup stocks, dried beans, and whole grains.

Day 1

BREAKFAST
Bring to boil in small saucepan:
$1\frac{1}{4}$ cups water

Stir in and cook, covered, about 90 minutes:
  ¼ cup rye berries
  ¼ cup fine wheat bran
Serve topped with:
  ½ cup milk

LUNCH
Stuff:
  1 sweet red pepper
with mixture of:
  ½ cup cut-up strawberries
  ½ cup cottage or ricotta cheese

DINNER
Bring to boil:
  1–2 cups Bone Stock
Stir in:
  1 tablespoon whole-grain corn grits
  1 tablespoon dried lima beans, presoaked
Simmer till beans and grits are tender, then add:
  1 tablespoon cubed beef or pork browned in 1 teaspoon oil
    or butter

SNACK
  Leftover soup from dinner

Day 2
BREAKFAST
Bring to boil in small saucepan:
  ¾ cup water
Stir in and cook, covered, about 25 minutes:
  ¼ cup whole-grain corn meal that has been mixed with ½
    cup cold water
  1 tablespoon fine wheat bran or oat bran
Stir frequently to prevent sticking. Serve topped with:
  ½ cup milk

LUNCH
Finger foods, as much as you want:
>Cauliflower pieces
>Broccoli pieces
>Sweet green and red pepper rings
>Onion rings

Accompany with:
>Low- or No-Calorie Salad Dressing

DINNER
Top:
>2 cups veal stock prepared from Bone Stock recipe, jellied, cold

with:
>1 tablespoon slivered almonds
>1 slice lemon

Serve with:
>Your choice of vegetables from the High-Potassium Foods list, steamed

SNACK
>1–2 cups Basic High-Potassium Soup

Day 3

BREAKFAST
Bring to boil in small saucepan:
>1¼ cups water

Stir in and cook, covered, about 45 minutes:
>¼ cup millet
>¼ cup fine wheat or oat bran

Serve topped with:
>½ cup milk

LUNCH
Stuff:
>Celery sticks

with:
>½ cup laban (thick yogurt) mixed with horseradish to taste

DINNER
Bring to boil in large saucepan:
    2–3 cups Bone Stock prepared with lamb bones
*Add and simmer slowly until done (about 45 minutes; 20
    minutes in pressure cooker):*
    1 tablespoon whole barley
Then add:
    1 tablespoon soybeans, cooked
    2 tablespoons tomato paste (unsalted)
    1 tablespoon minced lamb, browned in 1 teaspoon butter
    2–4 cups vegetables from the High-Potassium Foods list,
        chopped as coarse or as fine as you like
Continue simmering till vegetables are tender.

SNACK
    Leftover soup from dinner

Day 4
BREAKFAST
Mix together:
    ¼ cup fine wheat bran
    ¼ cup toasted wheat germ
    ½ cup hot milk
Allow to stand several minutes, till milk is absorbed.

LUNCH
Toss together:
    2 cups shredded kale (more or less)
    ½–1 red onion, sliced thin
    1 teaspoon caraway seed
    Low- or No-Calorie Salad Dressing

DINNER
Bring to simmer:
    2–4 cups veal stock prepared from Bone Stock recipe
Add and simmer 2 minutes:
    1–2 cups vegetables from High-Potassium Foods list, very
        thinly sliced

Remove from heat and add in a thin stream while continuing to stir:
    1 egg, beaten
Serve immediately.

SNACK
    Leftover soup from dinner

Day 5

BREAKFAST
Bring to boil in small saucepan:
    1¼ cups water
Stir in and cook, covered, about 90 minutes:
    ¼ cup wheat berries
    ¼ cup fine wheat or oat bran
Serve topped with:
    ½ cup milk

LUNCH
    Asparagus (unlimited), raw or lightly steamed
    1 egg, hard-boiled and sliced, or soft-boiled
    Low- or No-Calorie Salad Dressing

DINNER
Bring to boil in large saucepan:
    2–4 cups Bone Stock prepared with beef bones
Add:
    1 tablespoon whole barley
    1 tablespoon dried black beans, presoaked
    1–4 cloves garlic, minced
    ½ onion, sliced
Simmer till barley and beans are almost done, then add:
    2–4 cups vegetables from High-Potassium Foods list, cut up
    1 rib celery, sliced
    ½ carrot, sliced
Continue cooking till vegetables are done to your liking. Stir in:
    ⅛ pound liver, in very thin slivers
Turn off heat immediately and serve.

SNACK
  Leftover soup from dinner

Day 6

BREAKFAST
Bring to boil in small saucepan:
  1 cup water
Stir in and cook, covered, about 10 minutes:
  ¼ cup oatmeal
  ¼ cup fine wheat bran or rice bran
Serve topped with:
  ½ cup milk

LUNCH
Stuff:
  1 green pepper
with mixture of:
  ½ cup cottage or ricotta cheese
  ½ cup chopped cooked shrimp
  Curry powder to taste

DINNER
Bring to boil:
  2–4 cups chicken stock prepared from Bone Stock recipe
Stir in:
  1 tablespoon raw brown rice
Cover and simmer about 45 minutes; when done add:
  1 ounce tofu
  3 raw shrimp, peeled and deveined
  1 scallion, sliced
  Celery leaves, chopped (optional)
Simmer 2–3 minutes longer, just until shrimp are done.

SNACK
  Leftover soup from dinner

Day 7
BREAKFAST
Bring to boil in small saucepan:
    1½ cups water
Stir in and cook, covered, about 70 minutes:
    ¼ cup whole barley
    ¼ cup fine wheat bran or rice bran
Serve topped with:
    ½ cup milk

LUNCH
Toss together:
    2–4 cups fresh spinach
    Sliced mushrooms, as much as you want
    1 teaspoon nuts or seeds
    Low- or No-Calorie Salad Dressing

DINNER
Combine and bring to boil:
    2–4 cups veal stock prepared from Bone Stock recipe
    2 cups zucchini, sliced, shredded, or pureed
    2–6 cloves garlic, minced
Simmer till done, then add:
    1 teaspoon fruity olive oil

SNACK
    Leftover soup from dinner

Day 8
BREAKFAST
Bring to boil in small saucepan:
    1½ cups water
Stir in and cook, covered, about 70 minutes:
    ¼ cup whole barley
    ¼ cup fine wheat bran or rice bran
Serve topped with:
    ½ cup milk

LUNCH
    2–4 cups any vegetables from High-Potassium Foods list
    Low-or No-Calorie Salad Dressing

DINNER
Steam until just tender:
    2–4 cups broccoli and cauliflower
Spread immediately with:
    ¼ cup plain yogurt mixed with 1 teaspoon to 2 tablespoons
        horseradish
or:
    ¼ cup cottage cheese mixed with 1 teaspoon blue,
        roquefort, or Parmesan cheese

SNACK
    1–2 cups Basic High-Potassium Soup prepared with Bone
        Stock base

Day 9
BREAKFAST
Combine:
    ¼ cup toasted wheat germ
    ¼ cup fine wheat bran
    ¼ cup hot water, or enough to thicken
Serve topped with:
    ½ cup milk

LUNCH
Stir together:
    1–2 cucumbers, sliced very thin
    1 cup yogurt
    Dill to taste
    Minced garlic to taste

DINNER
Bring to boil:
    2–4 cups chicken stock prepared from Bone Stock recipe
Add and simmer till tender:
    1–2 cups asparagus pieces

Stir in:
> ¼ pound veal cut into matchstick slivers and browned in 1
> teaspoon olive oil or butter

Serve immediately.

SNACK
> Leftover soup from dinner

Day 10
BREAKFAST
Bring to boil in small saucepan:
> 1½ cups water

Stir in and cook, covered, about 20 minutes:
> ¼ cup whole rolled oats
> ¼ cup fine wheat, oat, or rice bran

Serve topped with:
> ½ cup milk

LUNCH
Toss together:
> 1 kohlrabi, peeled and shredded
> 1 zucchini, shredded
> 1 teaspoon dark sesame oil

DINNER
Heat together gently:
> 6 oysters
> 1 teaspoon butter

Then add:
> 1 cup milk

Heat and top with freshly ground black pepper. Serve with:
> Your choice of vegetables from High-Potassium Foods list
> Low- or No-Calorie Salad Dressing

SNACK
> 1–2 cups Basic High-Potassium Soup prepared with Bone
> Stock base

Nutrient Analysis

These tables show the average daily nutrients supplied by the Regularity Diet so you can see how they compare with standard recommendations. Figures include the nutrients provided by the basic diet as listed in the daily menus, and the nutrients supplied if my recommendation to use the High-Nutrient Soup as a supplement is followed. The averages are based on the ten-day total for each nutrient, and the figures have been rounded off. (For a fuller discussion of what the figures mean, turn to page 49.)

The Regularity Diet:
Meeting Your Needs for Nutrients Having Established RDA *

	RDA		Daily Average Supplied by Diet	
Nutrient	Woman Aged 23–50	Man Aged 23–50	Basic Diet, No Additions	Total with Soup Addition
Vitamin A	4000 IU	5000 IU	7495 IU	17,535 IU
Vitamin B-1	1.0 mg	1.4 mg	0.84 mg	1.4 mg
Vitamin B-2	1.2 mg	1.6 mg	1.3 mg	2.3 mg
Vitamin B-3	13 mg	18 mg	9.9 mg	16.7 mg
Vitamin B-6	2.0 mg	2.2 mg	1.0 mg	2.0 mg
Vitamin B-12	3.0 mcg	3.0 mcg	7.8 mcg	12.3 mcg
Vitamin C	60 mg	60 mg	194 mg	414 mg
Calcium	800 mg	800 mg	536 mg	944 mg
Vitamin D†	200 IU	200 IU	—	—
Vitamin E	11.9 IU	14.9 IU	10.3 IU	15.7 IU
Folacin	400 mcg	400 mcg	268 mcg	597 mcg
Iodine†	150 mcg	150 mcg	—	—
Iron	18 mg	10 mg	11.2 mg	19 mg
Magnesium	300 mg	350 mg	260 mg	465 mg
Phosphorus	800 mg	800 mg	890 mg	1265 mg
Protein	44 gm	56 gm	34.8 gm	50 gm
Zinc	15 mg	15 mg	14 mg	19.3 mg

Nutrient values of daily menus were calculated with Health-Aide nutrition software, Programming Technology Corporation, San Rafael, California, 1982.

* The Recommended Dietary Allowances (RDA) are taken from Commmittee on Dietary Allowances, Food and Nutrition Board, *Recommended Dietary Allowances* (ninth revised edition), Washington, D.C. Complete information for age groups other than those listed here, and for pregnant or lactating women, may be found on page 291.

† Nutrient values for vitamin D and iodine are indeterminate, but it is very unlikely that anyone will get less than the full RDA daily if milk or fish is included in the diet.

gm = gram   IU = international unit   mcg = microgram   mg = milligram

The Regularity Diet: Other Important Nutritional Needs

Nutrient	Recommendation*	Daily Average Supplied by Diet		Comment†
		Basic Diet, No Additions	Total with Soup Addition	
Calories	Varies	504	749	Add treats or needs or both to bring calories to desired level
Carbohydrates	Approximately 58% total calories	115 gm	165 gm	Carbohydrates = about 88% daily calories; you may want to add protein foods
Crude Fiber	6 gm or more	6 gm	12.5 gm	Strain the soup if it has too much roughage for you
Potassium	1875–5625 mg	2043 mg	4364 mg	Stay on the high side
All Fats‡	Not to exceed 30% total calories	13 gm	15.1 gm	⎫ Fats = 18% daily calories (6% saturated, 6% monounsaturated, 1.5% polyunsaturated)
Saturated	Approximately 10% total calories	4.5 gm	4.6 gm	
Monounsaturated	Approximately 10% total calories	4.3 gm	4.6 gm	
Polyunsaturated	Approximately 10% total calories	1.2 gm	1.2 gm	⎭
Cholesterol	300 mg maximum	121 mg	131 mg	Keep on the low side
Sodium	1100–3300 mg maximum	376 mg	662 mg	Keep on the low side
Sugar	Not to exceed 10% total calories	1 gm	1 gm	Sugar = less than 1% daily calories

Nutrient values of daily menus were calculated with Health-Aide nutrition software, Programming Technology Corporation, San Rafael, California, 1982.

* Nutrient Recommendations regarding carbohydrates, fats, cholesterol, and sugar are part of the Dietary Goals for the United States, prepared by the Senate Select Committee on Nutrition and Human Needs, 1977. Other recommendations are broad guidelines as reported in *Recommended Dietary Allowances.*

† Percentages are based on total with soup addition.

‡ Because values are not available for some minor fatty acids, the amounts listed in each group do not add up to the total for all fats.

Customizing the Diet

CALCULATING CALORIE NEEDS

1. Enter here your daily calorie needs or goals: _____
   (Use the table on page 50, or follow the guidelines in
   Chapter 12 for finding your personal balance. Remember, for best health results, women should generally consume no fewer than 1200 calories daily, and
   men no fewer than 1500, for any extended period of
   time.)
2. This is the average daily number of calories in the
   basic diet, without additions: 504
3. Subtract step 2 from step 1 to learn how many additional calories daily you will require, on average: _____

FILLING YOUR NEEDS: SOME SUGGESTIONS

1. As shown in the nutrient analysis tables, adding *half* the High-
   Nutrient Soup recipe (see page 228) *daily* completes most nutritional requirements while adding just 245 calories per day.
   If you choose not to add the High-Nutrient Soup, the lists in
   Food Sources of Major Nutrients, Chapter 17, will help you
   select foods to meet your nutritional needs. You could, for
   example, forgo the extra soup and instead add these foods to
   the daily diet:

   ½ pound raw kale
   1 banana or other B-6 food
   4 ounces tuna, turkey, or other protein source
   1 large oyster or other zinc source

   To meet iron requirements, women could have more oysters
   daily or could add ½ pound raw chard or other iron-rich food.
2. Even with the soup addition, men will need to make sure they
   get enough vitamins B-3 and B-6 and protein. Adding 1 pound
   of kale, 3 or 4 bananas, and three servings of tuna during the
   course of the ten days would cover these requirements.
3. Once you are sure your nutrient needs are taken care of, you
   can add other foods you like to bring your calorie intake to the
   desired level. The lists in Chapter 14 and Chapter 17 will help
   you make good choices.

How Is the Diet Going?

The checklists and chart will help you keep track of how you're feeling and how you're doing on this diet. Paying close attention to your body's signals may help you determine whether this is the diet for you.

The Regularity Diet:
Daily Checklist of Negative and Positive Factors

	DAY									
NEGATIVE FACTORS	1	2	3	4	5	6	7	8	9	10
Constipated										
Diarrhea										
Sleepless										
Irritable										
Itchy										
Sneezing										
Hungry										
Headache										
Blackout										
Gas										
Heartburn										
Bloat										
Weakness										
Fatigue										
Nervous										
Anxious										
Tremors										

POSITIVE FACTORS

Bowel movement*										
Sleeping well										
Stomach satisfied										
Alert, clear-headed										
Feel strong										
Lively										

* 1–3 times/day with regular, well-formed stool

The Regularity Diet:
Daily Weight Change Chart

The horizontal line through the middle of the chart represents your starting weight (Day 1). Each day, mark a new point to show how your weight is changing (or not) as the diet progresses. Draw a line from point to point to chart your weight change.

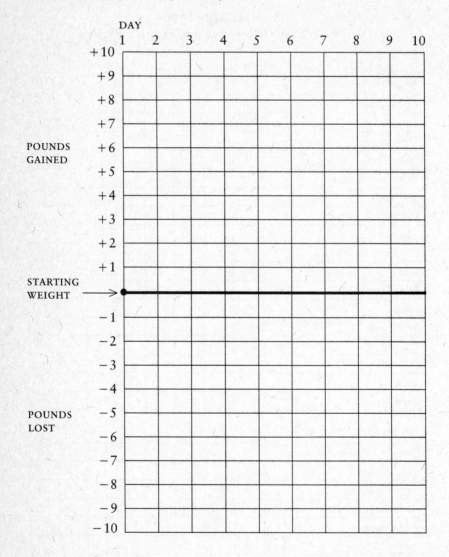

Beating Laxatives and Suppositories

Constipation is a serious problem in the United States and in any other country where refined foods are eaten to excess. It is often the case, on such a diet, that you will find that you are not losing weight because you did not have a bowel movement when you should. (A normal stool can easily weigh from ½ pound to 1½ pounds.) Many people, because of inadequate diets, take laxatives or use suppositories on a daily basis — sometimes for years, often for almost an entire lifetime.

The real reason we turn to such remedies is lack of food elements that are essential to healthy living: sufficient bulk, sufficient water, sufficient roughage, sufficient fats, sufficient oils, sufficient magnesium and potassium, and sufficient physical activity. It makes no difference how long you may have been using laxatives or suppositories. There are few people who cannot beat the habit.

How the Colon Works

In the digestive process helpful chemicals are *added* to the food you've ingested and nutrients taken away, in the mouth, the stomach, the small intestine, and the large intestine. (The largest amount of nutrient *retrieval* seems to be from the small intestine.) The colon, or large intestine, has rings of smooth muscle around it by which it moves the contents (the food you have eaten) through. As the food is moved along, water and other substances in it are transported back to the circulation through the intestinal walls, in this way condensing the mass in the colon and hardening the stool. The milking action of the gut is called peristalsis.

There is a race between the pulling of fluids from the stool back into the body and the peristalsis pushing the stool along. So having the stool in the body too long leads to hard, relatively dry stools that are difficult to pass. Fiber retains water in the stool and keeps it soft and bulky, with the usual results being easy passage.

When peristalsis slows down (lack of potassium can cause this), the contents of the colon are very difficult to move along. When the colon muscles contract strongly and will not relax (spasms), it is often for lack of magnesium, which can be responsible for spasms in any muscle, anywhere in the body. If only high-protein or soft, refined foods are eaten, there is little bulk or roughage for the colon to contract against. It is much harder for the colon to move along a pencil-thin mass than a larger, bulky mass. (When the toothpaste tube is almost empty, how hard is it to get the toothpaste out? When the tube is full, it takes a lot less effort to extrude the paste. The principle is the same.)

How to Become Unconstipated

If you want to have a normal-sized, easy-to-pass movement, one to three times a day, you needn't increase your intake of calories, but the bulk, roughage, and other nutrients *must be increased*. It is not healthy to carry around garbage in your gut, where it gets drier and drier and ferments more and more. But this is common on a diet high in foods without roughage or a poor high-protein diet. A diet high in potassium-rich foods (unrefined foods such as bran, nuts and seeds, vegetables, and fruits are all naturally high in potassium and magnesium) is essential to help the muscles around the colon to contract strongly and to have enough bulk to contract against. You can satisfy *all* the elements your body needs to pass trouble-free stools by eating unrefined fruits and vegetables and whole grains, nuts, and seeds. (If these are the foods that relieve constipation, why did we ever get started eating refined foods?)

Fresh fruits and vegetables provide some roughage and bulk and also provide potassium and magnesium. For persons with digestive problems it is safer to start with cooked fruits and vegetables and very gradually move to small amounts of foods with more roughage or to raw foods. Seeds and nuts are a better source of roughage, have potassium and magnesium, and are high in oils, which are often helpful to those with constipation.

Most people I have worked with recover the ability to pass a trouble-free stool by using nuts and seeds as their daily cereal (see the various cereal recipes in Chapter 14). Bran and the outer coverings of rice and other grains provide more *roughage* than fruits, vegetables, or nuts and seeds but are sometimes too rough to be usable by those who have made the digestive tract delicate with the use of soft foods. For that reason brans should be introduced into the diet in small amounts and increased very gradually. Fine (finely ground) brans of oats, corn, rice, or wheat are better for those with delicate digestive tracts than the rougher whole form. Bran seems to act like a sponge, picking up fluids and holding onto them, keeping the stool soft. This helps maintain a bulkiness that allows the stool to be passed along easily.

Is Constipation So Bad?

Hemorrhoids are a bad enough consequence of constipation to deal with. There are worse. A hard stool has literally caused many people to die on the toilet. Heavy straining while holding the breath pushes the blood pressure up and causes blood vessels to break. You may have seen women who in childbirth suddenly acquire broken blood vessels in the legs (and in the face; I watched it happen at one birth I attended). These are caused mainly from pushing hard without breathing out at the same time to relieve some of the pressure. You could, while straining because of constipation, break weakened blood vessels not only in your face or legs but in your head as well (perhaps even causing a stroke!). It is important to prevent ever having to push hard again to have a bowel movement. It is neither natural nor necessary.

Add bulk, roughage, water, oils, magnesium, and potassium to your diet till you have control of the texture of your stool.

I Ate That Way for a Week and It's Not Working

Most people can modify their eating habits and retrain their bowel functions, but the changes must be made gradually.

The First Week. If you take laxatives, continue to take them every day. Eat vegetables and fruits, raw or cooked, and whole grains and unroasted nuts and seeds daily. You must add bulk or roughage and other helpful nutrients to aid your digestive tract.

The Second Week. Continue to eat the same foods but take the laxative only every other day. Before getting out of bed on the day you don't take a laxative, roll onto your back, bend your knees with your feet flat on the bed, and loosely, using your belly muscles, "blop" your belly in and out, 20 to 50 times. This helps to get the peristalsis (the wavelike movements of the colon) speeded up. After you get out of bed have a full glass of hot water (with half a lemon squeezed into it if you want) and then a bran cereal or a nuts and seeds cereal, maybe with fresh fruit added or blackstrap molasses for a little insurance. (Blackstrap is well known for its ability to ease the movement of bowels — and without roughage! It is high in iron, potassium, magnesium, and calcium.) During the rest of the day either use the Regularity Diet or choose your foods from the lists of high-fiber, high-potassium, or high-magnesium foods in Chapter 17. Don't worry if you don't always have a bowel movement on these in-between days. If you've been taking laxatives for a long time, your body may need a little while to learn the new routine. Give it time.

The Third Week. Try two days off laxatives, doing your "belly bloppers," and one day on laxatives. Keep up your intake of the useful foods. If you get lazy about eating unrefined foods at this stage, you may upset the whole system and have to start over. Keep right with it. It's a good feeling to have your body doing its own work again and certainly much healthier for you.

The Fourth Week. Take a laxative only one or two days and only if you feel your body is a little slow in adjusting to doing its own work. If you do feel your body is responding slowly, continue to do the belly bloppers, even doing them every day, in the morning and at night.

Kicking the laxative habit is worth the work involved. There are lots of bonuses: you can improve your diet and so become healthier, be more comfortable, save money, and be free of laxatives!

❧ 6 ❧

The Raw Diet

For well over a hundred years raw food diets have been touted for their benefits to our health. What do we know about them? Humans cook food to change its taste, to soften it, to increase digestibility, and, as we now know, to rid it of harmful bacteria and parasites. The advantages of raw foods are not only that the tastes are quite as interesting as when they are cooked, but that they also promote longer chewing time, which is both good for the gums and teeth and helps to limit how much is eaten at a meal. In addition, the salivary enzymes get more chance to work, and the digestive process is made easier when foods have been ground up by chewing.

The Raw Diet is one variation on eating that has appealed to many people over the years. The Japanese eat much of their food raw, even seaweed and fish. Raw fish is not just edible, it is also delicious, as the Japanese and other cultures have known for years.

Unfortunately, we have now polluted our lakes and rivers so badly that you may become very ill if you eat freshwater fish raw or even cooked. Ocean fish, on the other hand, caught at least three to five miles offshore (to avoid the known polluted areas) are still generally safe. You need a fish market that you can trust implicitly. Shellfish gathered too close to shore can carry disease, so don't eat these raw, and don't trust the usual cooking methods to kill disease germs either. (It takes an unbelievably long time to fry clams in such a way as to guarantee no hepatitis virus.) And of course, any time you have any doubts about the freshness or cleanliness of your raw fish, cooking is safer.

All the fruits and vegetables used in the Raw Diet are best bought fresh and locally grown. Foods that are shipped long distances are often picked unripe for ease in shipping, then have chemicals used on them to prevent ripening in transit, and finally are ripened with more chemicals before they are placed on the shelves. Buy carefully and wash them well.

The Raw Diet is excellent for some of us. But no diet is good for everyone. There are good reasons why, for many people, the Raw Diet would not be acceptable. There are some who cannot digest raw foods. Chunks or shreds may come through in the stool. The raw food in whole form may give you gas, diarrhea, or just upset your system generally. Some people with sensitive colons cannot tolerate roughage. Others are allergic to certain raw plant food, and yet others can't chew, for lack of proper alignment of teeth or even lack of teeth. Individuals who would have trouble chewing raw foods may do very well if the foods are put through a blender or made into juice, which removes the roughage altogether. I have seen very ill people who did well on foods — both fruits and vegetables — that had been put through a juicer. Nevertheless, for one reason or another, many people will want their vegetables and even their fruits cooked, regardless of the various ways in which some of the vitamins and minerals are lost directly or indirectly by cooking.

 Every diet you try must fit *you!* No matter how good it is to look at or taste, it must fit *you, your* capabilities, *your* digestion, and *your* likes and dislikes.

But certainly with reasonably pure food sources the Raw Diet is one of the prettiest and easiest of the diets. It requires no cooking and it retains the bright and beautiful colors of the fresh fruits and vegetables.

Shopping List

A bullet (•) indicates the specific foods called for in the daily menus. The other listed foods would be good additions to the core diet.

SEAFOOD (same-day fresh, not frozen)
fish (ocean fish only)
• bass
• mackerel
• swordfish
• tuna
shellfish (from *clean* sources)
• clams
• oysters
• scallops
sea urchins
• shrimp

MEATS
• liver (any kind)

DAIRY PRODUCTS (all lowfat, no added salt or sugar; cultured if available)*
• buttermilk
cheeses
• cheddar cheese
• cottage cheese
• ricotta cheese
• eggs
• laban (thickened yogurt)
sweet acidophilus milk
• yogurt

VEGETABLES
• alfalfa sprouts
• avocado
• broccoli
• cabbage (all kinds)
• carrots
• cauliflower
• celery
chili peppers
• cucumbers
• garlic
• kale
• lettuce, butterhead and looseleaf
• onions, white
• parsley
• peppers, sweet green and red
• scallions
sprouts, various
• tomatoes
• watercress
• zucchini

FRUITS
• apricots, fresh or dried
• blueberries
• cantaloupe
grapefruit
• honeydew melon
• lemons
• mango
• oranges

• papaya
• peaches, fresh or dried
• pineapple
• plums
• prunes, dried
raspberries
• strawberries
• watermelon

NUTS, SEEDS, AND GRAINS (unroasted, unsalted)
• almonds
Brazil nuts
• nuts (all varieties)
• oat bran
• pecans
• pumpkin seeds
• seeds (all varieties)
sesame seeds
• sunflower seeds
• wheat bran (fine)

OTHER
• carrot juice
• chives
• dark sesame oil
• dill
• fresh basil
• olive oil
• wasabi (Japanese horseradish)

* Unless you have an impeccable source, do not use raw milk; use pasteurized products only.

Daily Menus

The basic recipes and food lists referred to in the menus may be
found in Chapter 14.

Day 1
BREAKFAST
>½ mango
>½ cup yogurt

LUNCH
>¼ cup your choice from Nuts and Seeds list
>1 fresh peach *or* 2 dried halves

DINNER
Toss together:
>⅛ pound tiny, sweet raw shrimp
>⅛ pound raw scallops, tiny or sliced
>Dill
>Chives
>10 or more leaves butterhead lettuce
>½ cup watercress
>Low- or No-Calorie Salad Dressing

SNACK
Put through juicer for fresh vegetable juice:
>3 carrots
>1 rib celery

Day 2
BREAKFAST
Mix in blender:
>½ papaya, cut up
>¼ cup fine oat or wheat bran
>1 cup buttermilk

LUNCH
>6 raw oysters
>Large dark green salad
>Low- or No-Calorie Salad Dressing

DINNER
> ½ cup cottage or ricotta cheese
> Finger salad: carrots, sweet green peppers, cucumbers
> ½ peach
> ⅛ cantaloupe

SNACK
> ¼ cup pecans and pumpkin seeds

Day 3
BREAKFAST
> ¼ cup your choice from Nuts and Seeds list
> 1 cup yogurt

LUNCH
> 6 raw clams
> Finger salad: carrots, zucchini, cucumbers, sweet red
> > peppers
> Low- or No-Calorie Salad Dressing or dip if you want

DINNER
> 1 cup cottage or ricotta cheese, with fresh herbs
> Large green salad *or* steamed vegetables from the High-
> > Potassium Foods list
> Low- or No-Calorie Salad Dressing if you want

SNACK
> ¼ fresh pineapple cut in sticks or chunks

Day 4
BREAKFAST
Stir together:
> ½ cantaloupe, cut up
> 1 cup yogurt

LUNCH
> ⅛ pound cheddar cheese, cut into small pieces
> 1 cup fresh strawberries

DINNER
   ½ pound altogether of raw bass, scallops, tuna
   Small amount wasabi (Japanese horseradish), if desired
Serve with a salad made by mixing together:
   1 cup shredded zucchini and cucumbers
   2 tablespoons yogurt seasoned to taste with dill and garlic *or*
      a few drops dark sesame oil

SNACK
   2 fresh apricots *or* 4 dried halves

Day 5
BREAKFAST
Spoon:
   ¼ fresh pineapple, crushed
over:
   1 cup yogurt

LUNCH
Serve on half shell:
   3 raw clams
   3 raw oysters
Accompany with:
   ¼ honeydew melon

DINNER
Make a blender soup. First whirl together until smooth:
   2 tomatoes
   ¼ small white onion
   ⅛ lemon, with peel
Then add the following vegetables, coarsely chopped:
   ½ green pepper
   ¼ cucumber
   1 scallion
   Few sprigs parsley, minced
   Few leaves fresh basil, cut up
   Anything else you like from the High-Potassium Foods list

SNACK
   ¼ cup almonds

Day 6

BREAKFAST
Mix together:
    ¼ cup your choice from Nuts and Seeds list, ground
    ½ cup blueberries
    ½ cup yogurt

LUNCH
Serve:
    ¼ pound very thin slices liver browned in 1 teaspoon olive
        oil (see note)
on a bed of:
    1 chopped scallion
    1 cup alfalfa sprouts (or as much as you want)
*Note: Some Armenian restaurants serve chunks of raw liver, raw
onion, and raw tomato with a little olive oil and pita bread.*

DINNER
Serve on half shell:
    3 raw clams
    3 raw oysters
Accompany with a salad of:
    ½ avocado
    Watercress
    Low- or No-Calorie Salad Dressing

SNACK
Prepare slices of fresh vegetables, such as:
    Sweet red peppers, celery, and others
Dip into:
    ½ cup spiced laban or yogurt

Day 7

BREAKFAST
    ¹⁄₁₀ honeydew melon (fresh mint, lemon juice, or lime juice is
        great with honeydew)
    1 cup cottage or ricotta cheese

LUNCH
Salad bar:
  Broccoli
  Sweet red or green peppers
  Cauliflower
  Onions
  Alfalfa sprouts
Carry your salad dressing if you're going to be out.

DINNER
  ¼ pound altogether of mackerel, swordfish, or scallops
    (whatever is freshest or your favorite)
  Wasabi (if you choose)
  ½ papaya

SNACK
Mix together in blender:
  1 orange, thinly peeled and cut up (retain as much of the
    white part of the peel as you can)
  1 raw egg

Day 8
BREAKFAST
  ½ grapefruit
  ¼ cup your choice from Nuts and Seeds list

LUNCH
  1 cup yogurt
  1 peach

DINNER
  ½ cup cottage or ricotta cheese with herbs
  ½ avocado
  Large green salad
  Low- or No-Calorie Salad Dressing

SNACK
  ¼ honeydew melon (or equivalent-sized wedge of
    watermelon)

Day 9
BREAKFAST
Put through juicer for fresh vegetable juice:
    3 carrots
    1 green pepper
    1 rib celery
Accompany with:
    ¼ cup sunflower and pumpkin seeds

LUNCH
    ¼ pound mixed shrimp (use small, sweet ones), sea urchin,
        tuna
    Wasabi (if you like)
    Large green salad from the High-Potassium Foods list
    Low- or No-Calorie Salad Dressing

DINNER
Enjoy as finger foods:
    ⅛ pound cheddar cheese
    ⅛ fresh pineapple
    ⅛ honeydew melon

SNACK
Mix together:
    ¼ cup yogurt
    1 cucumber, chopped
    Minced garlic
    Dill

Day 10
BREAKFAST
Stir together:
    ½ cup berries (your choice)
    1 cup yogurt

LUNCH
    ⅛ pound cheddar cheese, cut up as finger food
    Large sprout salad or other salad
    Low- or No-Calorie Salad Dressing

DINNER
Serve on half shell:
    6 raw oysters
Accompany with a salad of:
    1 cup shredded kale
    1 cup shredded red or white cabbage
    Any other vegetable you like from the High-Potassium
        Foods list
    ½ onion, thinly sliced in rings
    Low- or No-Calorie Salad Dressing

SNACK
    4 fresh plums or prunes

Nutrient Analysis

These tables show the average daily nutrients supplied by the Raw Diet so you can see how they compare with standard recommendations. Figures include the nutrients provided by the basic diet as listed in the daily menus, and the nutrients supplied if my recommendation to use the High-Nutrient Soup as a supplement is followed. The averages are based on the ten-day total for each nutrient, and the figures have been rounded off. (For a fuller discussion of what the figures mean, turn to page 49.)

The Raw Diet:
Meeting Your Needs for Nutrients Having Established RDA *

	RDA		Daily Average Supplied by Diet	
Nutrient	Woman Aged 23–50	Man Aged 23–50	Basic Diet, No Additions	Total with Soup Addition
Vitamin A	4000 IU	5000 IU	27,200 IU	37,240 IU
Vitamin B-1	1.0 mg	1.4 mg	0.84 mg	1.4 mg
Vitamin B-2	1.2 mg	1.6 mg	2.1 mg	3.1 mg
Vitamin B-3	13 mg	18 mg	12.4 mg	19.2 mg
Vitamin B-6	2.0 mg	2.2 mg	1.2 mg	2.2 mg
Vitamin B-12	3.0 mcg	3.0 mcg	25.9 mcg	30.4 mcg
Vitamin C	60 mg	60 mg	199 mg	419 mg
Calcium	800 mg	800 mg	1008 mg	1416 mg
Vitamin D†	200 IU	200 IU	—	—
Vitamin E	11.9 IU	14.9 IU	13.5 IU	18.9 IU
Folacin	400 mcg	400 mcg	244 mcg	573 mcg
Iodine†	150 mcg	150 mcg	—	—
Iron	18 mg	10 mg	14.8 mg	22.6 mg
Magnesium	300 mg	350 mg	240 mg	445 mg
Phosphorus	800 mg	800 mg	864 mg	1239 mg
Protein	44 gm	56 gm	57.2 gm	72.5 gm
Zinc	15 mg	15 mg	30 mg	35.3 mg

Nutrient values of daily menus were calculated with Health-Aide nutrition software, Programming Technology Corporation, San Rafael, California, 1982.

* The Recommended Dietary Allowances (RDA) are taken from Committee on Dietary Allowances, Food and Nutrition Board, *Recommended Dietary Allowances* (ninth revised edition), Washington, D.C. Complete information for age groups other than those listed here, and for pregnant or lactating women, may be found on page 291.

† Nutrient values for vitamin D and iodine are indeterminate, but it is very unlikely that anyone will get less than the full RDA daily if milk or fish is included in the diet.

gm = gram   IU = international unit   mcg = microgram   mg = milligram

The Raw Diet: Other Important Nutritional Needs

Nutrient	Recommendation*	Daily Average Supplied by Diet		Comment†
		Basic Diet, No Additions	Total with Soup Addition	
Calories	Varies	852	1097	Add treats or needs or both to bring calories to desired level
Carbohydrates	Approximately 58% total calories	90 gm	140 gm	Carbohydrates = about 51% daily calories
Crude Fiber	6 gm or more	7 gm	13.5 gm	Strain the soup if it has too much roughage for you
Potassium	1875–5625 mg	2834 mg	5155 mg	Stay on the high side
All Fats‡	Not to exceed 30% total calories	34 gm	36.1 gm	} Fats = 30% daily calories (7.5% saturated, 9.3% monounsaturated, 5% polyunsaturated)
Saturated	Approximately 10% total calories	9 gm	9.1 gm	
Monounsaturated	Approximately 10% total calories	11 gm	11.3 gm	
Polyunsaturated	Approximately 10% total calories	6 gm	6 gm	
Cholesterol	300 mg maximum	146 mg	156 mg	Keep on the low side
Sodium	1100–3300 mg maximum	733 mg	1019 mg	Keep on the low side
Sugar	Not to exceed 10% total calories	0 gm	0 gm	

Nutrient values of daily menus were calculated with Health-Aide nutrition software, Programming Technology Corporation, San Rafael, California, 1982.

* Nutrient Recommendations regarding carbohydrates, fats, cholesterol, and sugar are part of the Dietary Goals for the United States, prepared by the Senate Select Committee on Nutrition and Human Needs, 1977. Other recommendations are broad guidelines as reported in *Recommended Dietary Allowances.*

† Percentages are based on total with soup addition.

‡ Because values are not available for some minor fatty acids, the amounts listed in each group do not add up to the total for all fats.

Customizing the Diet

CALCULATING CALORIE NEEDS

1. Enter here your daily calorie needs or goals: _____
   (Use the table on page 50, or follow the guidelines in Chapter 12 for finding your personal balance. Remember, for best health results, women should generally consume no fewer than 1200 calories daily, and men no fewer than 1500, for any extended period of time.)
2. This is the average daily number of calories in the basic diet, without additions: 852
3. Subtract step 2 from step 1 to learn how many additional calories daily you will require, on average: _____

FILLING YOUR NEEDS: SOME SUGGESTIONS

1. As shown in the nutrient analysis tables, adding *half* the High-Nutrient Soup recipe (see page 228) *daily* completes nutritional requirements while adding just 245 calories per day.
2. If you choose not to use the High-Nutrient Soup, the lists in Food Sources of Major Nutrients, Chapter 17, will help you select foods to meet your nutritional needs. You could, for example, forgo the soup and round out nutrient requirements by adding these foods to the daily diet:

   1 cup raw asparagus
   1 cup raw mushrooms
   1½ cups raw spinach
   ¼ cup wheat bran or wheat germ

   To meet iron requirements, women should also add 1 cup chopped parsley or other iron-rich food daily.
   To meet vitamin B-1 requirements, men should be sure to use the wheat germ daily or add 1 cup peas or other B-1 food.
3. Once you are sure your nutrient needs are taken care of, you can add other foods you like to bring your calorie intake to the desired level. The lists in Chapter 14 will help you make good choices. The balance of carbohydrates, protein, and fats in this diet is already good, so try to maintain that balance in the selections you make.

How Is the Diet Going?

The checklists and chart will help you keep track of how you're feeling and how you're doing on this diet. Paying close attention to your body's signals may help you determine whether this is the diet for you.

The Raw Diet:
Daily Checklist of Negative and Positive Factors

NEGATIVE FACTORS	DAY 1	2	3	4	5	6	7	8	9	10
Constipated										
Diarrhea										
Sleepless										
Irritable										
Itchy										
Sneezing										
Hungry										
Headache										
Blackout										
Gas										
Heartburn										
Bloat										
Weakness										
Fatigue										
Nervous										
Anxious										
Tremors										

POSITIVE FACTORS

Bowel movement*										
Sleeping well										
Stomach satisfied										
Alert, clear-headed										
Feel strong										
Lively										

* 1–3 times/day with regular, well-formed stool

The Raw Diet: Daily Weight Change Chart

The horizontal line through the middle of the chart represents your starting weight (Day 1). Each day, mark a new point to show how your weight is changing (or not) as the diet progresses. Draw a line from point to point to chart your weight change.

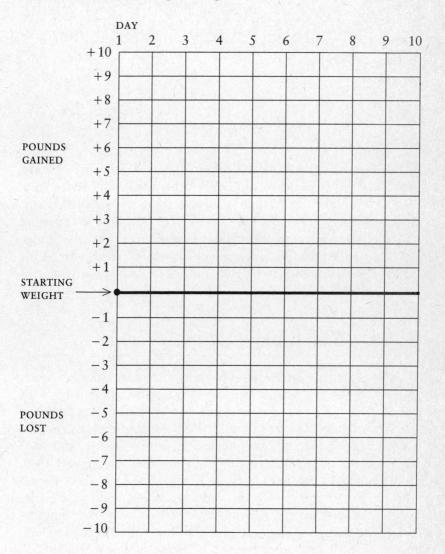

❧ 7 ❧

The Shine (Anti-Stress) Diet

For those of you who live between hammer and anvil, I have developed a diet to deal with a high-stress life. Under stress your body is not managing its input and output nearly as well as if you were relaxed. You can use up — or excrete — almost ten times as much calcium, magnesium, vitamins, and other nutrients under heavy stress as you do when under no stress. The Shine (Anti-Stress) Diet is designed to replace some of those lost nutrients.

Combating Day-to-day Stress

The idea of an anti-stress diet is to provide a smorgasbord of foods that are especially rich in nutrients. In my own experience with clients, I know of no diet that makes you look better and feel better so rapidly. The ability of the body to fight back against the ever-increasing load of contaminants in our air, water, and food has its limits. It seems reasonably obvious that we are very close to the edge. We can fight back to some degree for a short period of time, but we are already in overload and our bodies are giving way. How long we can fight off these toxins by further building our health is anybody's guess. For some of us, it's already too late, but others still have some leeway. How much leeway depends on genetics and general physical condition, and the amounts of pollutants presently attacking the system. There are probably people in your neighborhood right now who are suffering, some seriously, the effects of everyday pollutants in the environment. Many of the small discomforts for which people buy over-the-counter drugs are the result of allergies and sensitivities to environmental pollutants, some natural, many others unnatural.

There is much empirical evidence that the Shine Diet should help to make you healthier even if you are under heavy stress or have an illness or disease of any sort. (See the end of this chapter for a special note about this diet and progressive diseases.) The diet is not meant to cure anything. It is meant to build health so your body can fight its own battles. Of course, your doctor must be the source of dietary advice for any specific ailment you may have. *Don't* think this diet can take the place of a visit to your physician — he or she knows you best and can help you decide if this diet is all right for you to try.

The Shine Diet is a good premenstrual diet since menstrual periods are times of stress, when nutrients are being lost, sometimes disastrously fast. When supplemented with the Basic High-Potassium Soup or High-Nutrient Soup (Chapter 14), the diet is especially high in magnesium, which prevents menstrual cramps and also alleviates muscular cramps of other sorts, spasms, and trembling.

If you have a known allergy to a specific food in the diet plan, remove only that food, replace it with one equally nutrient-dense (consult the lists in the final chapter of the book), and continue with the diet, trying to stay as much with the suggested foods as you possibly can.

Another suggestion: If any foods on this diet upset your system, try them in a form other than the one that upset you. For example, try vegetables as juice instead of in whole form. In the case of dairy products, some kinds of milk cultures seem to prevent milk allergies in some otherwise allergic people while other cultures do not. Try small amounts of these foods spaced very far apart to see if there is a comfortable alternative for you. Milk is not the only source of calcium by a long shot. Try the suggested Basic High-Potassium Soup as a replacement. It is, in fact, a better source of calcium than milk, and few people are allergic to many vegetables.

Keep an Eye on Your Cholesterol Level

The foods in this diet include many against which you are tradi-
tionally warned, such as shellfish and organ meats, because of
their cholesterol content.

Many of us do not know our blood cholesterol levels. Some
people are prone to high blood cholesterol and some are not. If
you are one of the lucky ones whose blood cholesterol never rises
above 170 or 180, you can enjoy all the benefits of this diet with
not a worry in the world. Have your level checked. It is worthwhile if only to relieve your mind of one of the more justifiable
concerns of the moment.

If you *do* have an elevated cholesterol level, that is important to
know. You will find many stress-fighting factors (and absolutely
no cholesterol and few calories) in the Basic High-Potassium Soup,
which you can make a part of any diet plan you wish. It might be
worth experimenting with cod-liver oil and fatty fish such as halibut, salmon, mackerel, and others (a daily dose of cod-liver oil —
2000 international units vitamin A, 200 international units vitamin D — or one serving of fatty fish) to see if you can control
your own level of cholesterol. If these changes have not lowered
your cholesterol level by the end of a month, you might want to
consider going on a vegetarian diet, which for many people proves
to be a useful method of bringing down cholesterol levels. (This is
not to suggest that you should plunge into fancy vitamin supplements of D or any other vitamin. This book is based on getting
your vitamin D from the fish themselves or from the sun.)

When you have your cholesterol level under control, you may
want to try this diet, while at the same time taking cod-liver oil on
a daily basis. Common sense would indicate that you get regular
cholesterol checks for a while.

The 1986 American Heart Association recommendation limits
dietary cholesterol intake to 100 milligrams per 1000 calories and
no more than 300 milligrams per day. Since, as with salt, some
people are cholesterol-sensitive and some are not, this one diet
exceeds the recommended level by an enthusiastic amount — an
average 900 milligrams rather than 300. So again we stress that

you find your blood cholesterol level first to make sure that it is at 150, and we stress that if you have had to work to bring your level down to 150, then you should cut down on the use of all the high-cholesterol foods listed here — or use another of the diets.

The cholesterol occurs in the animal fats (and so does the saturated fat you are warned against). To help you in adjusting the diet, see the list of foods highest in cholesterol in the last chapter. For instance, a cup of cooked chicken livers gives you 883 milligrams of cholesterol, a half pound of cooked lobster 491 milligrams, and one large egg 274 milligrams.

From personal experience with students, I can tell you that those who can choose the Shine Diet really show the results in a luminescence of the skin, a brightness to the eye, and a higher level of energy.

Shopping List

A bullet (•) indicates the specific foods called for in the daily menus. The other listed foods would be good additions to the core diet.

SHELLFISH
- • clams
- conch
- • crab
- • lobster
- mussels
- • oysters
- prawns
- scallops
- • shrimp

MEATS (organ meats, any animal)
- gizzards
- • heart
- • kidneys
- • liver
- • sweetbreads

DAIRY PRODUCTS (all lowfat, no added salt or sugar; cultured if available)
- buttermilk
- cheeses
  - • cottage cheese
  - ricotta cheese
- • eggs
- laban (thickened yogurt)
- • milk
- • sweet acidophilus milk
- • yogurt

VEGETABLES
- • alfalfa sprouts
- • asparagus
- • bamboo shoots
- • bean sprouts
- • broccoli
- • Brussels sprouts
- • cabbage, Chinese, green, and red
- • carrots
- • cauliflower
- • cucumbers
- • dark leafy greens (all varieties)
- • endive
- • escarole
- • garlic
- • kale
- • lettuce, butterhead
- • mushrooms
- • onions, red and yellow
- • parsley
- • peppers, sweet green and red
- • spinach

FRUITS
- • apricots
- • cantaloupe
- • currants, dried
- • grapefruit
- mangos
- papaya
- • peaches
- • pineapple

NUTS, SEEDS, AND GRAINS (unroasted, unsalted)
- • caraway seeds
- • nuts (all varieties)
- • oat bran
- • seeds (all varieties)
- • wheat bran (fine)
- • wheat germ (toasted)

OILS, FATS (in order of preference)
- • olive oil
- • dark sesame oil
- • butter

OTHER
- • blackstrap molasses
- • carrot (or other vegetable) juice
- • fresh ginger
- • rice vinegar (or other vinegar)

Daily Menus
The basic recipes and food lists referred to in the menus may be found in Chapter 14.

Day 1
BREAKFAST
Simmer together:
> ¼ pound kidneys, sliced thin
> ¼ cup Bone Stock or Basic High-Potassium Soup broth
Season to taste. Serve with:
> ½ grapefruit

LUNCH
Stir together:
> ½ cup cubed cantaloupe
> ¼ cup your choice from Nuts and Seeds list, ground or whole
> 1 cup yogurt

DINNER
Steam and set aside:
> ¼ pound lobster meat
Then combine:
> 2 or more cups cut-up broccoli, cauliflower, and sweet red and green peppers (or other vegetables from the High-Potassium Foods list)
> ½ cup or more mushrooms, whole or sliced
Steam vegetables briefly, until crisp-tender. If desired, dress them lightly with:
> Low- or No-Calorie Salad Dressing
Serve with reserved lobster meat.

SNACK
Stir together:
> ½ cup warm sweet acidophilus milk
> 1 tablespoon blackstrap molasses

Day 2
BREAKFAST
Mix together:
   ¼ cup toasted wheat germ
   1 tablespoon fine wheat or oat bran
   ½ cup hot milk
Add:
   1 tablespoon blackstrap molasses *or* 1 serving from Fresh
      Fruits list

LUNCH
   ¼ pound shrimp, steamed *or* braised in 1 teaspoon butter
Serve with:
   Large green salad tossed with Low- or No-Calorie Salad
      Dressing
   1 cup fresh carrot juice (4–6 carrots if you make it yourself)

DINNER
Steam:
   ½ pound clams (1½ pounds in shell)
   ¼ pound mushrooms
in:
   1–2 cups chicken (or fish) stock prepared from Bone Stock
      recipe
Accompany with:
   1 cup shredded slaw vegetables (your choice) tossed
      with Low- or No-Calorie Salad Dressing

SNACK
   2 apricots

Day 3
BREAKFAST
   2 eggs, cooked any way you like (use no more than 1
      teaspoon butter or olive oil)

LUNCH
Serve on half shell:
   6 raw clams

Accompany with:
>Asparagus, as much as you want, raw or steamed
>Low- or No-Calorie Salad Dressing, if you want

DINNER
Prepare:
>¼ pound liver, thinly sliced
in one of the following ways:
>*gently braise over low heat in 1 teaspoon butter or olive oil*
>or *simmer in ½ cup Bone Stock or Basic High-Potassium Soup broth*
Accompany with:
>Large green salad, as much as you want, tossed with Low- or No-Calorie Salad Dressing

SNACK
>¼ cup your choice from Nuts and Seeds list

Day 4
BREAKFAST
Spoon:
>1 serving from Fresh Fruits list, cut up
>1 tablespoon toasted wheat germ
over:
>½ cup cottage cheese

LUNCH
Toss together:
>¼ cup crabmeat, steamed
>Large green salad
>Low- or No-Calorie Salad Dressing

DINNER
Preheat in wok or heavy skillet:
>1 teaspoon dark sesame oil
Toss in and stir-fry till lightly browned:
>1 clove garlic, minced
>1-inch piece fresh ginger, cut in matchsticks

Add and stir-fry till done to your liking:
>   ¼ pound beef heart or veal heart (or other organ meat),
>   cubed or cut in strips
>   ½ onion, sliced
>   ½ sweet pepper, sliced
>   Mushrooms, sliced
>   Parsley
>   Anything more you want from the High-Potassium Foods
>   list, shredded or sliced

SNACK
>   ½ grapefruit

Day 5
BREAKFAST
Sprinkle:
>   ¼ cup your choice from Nuts and Seeds list
>   1 teaspoon currants
over:
>   ½ cup yogurt

LUNCH
>   2 eggs, poached or boiled
>   1 serving from Fresh Fruits list

DINNER
>   1 cup strained broth from Basic High-Potassium Soup made
>   with Bone Stock base
Serve with:
>   ½ pound oysters and clams on half shell
and coleslaw made by tossing together:
>   ½ cup (or more) cabbage, red or green, sliced fine
>   ½ cup (or more) kale, sliced fine
>   ½ red onion, sliced fine
>   Caraway seeds
>   Low- or No-Calorie Salad Dressing

SNACK
>   1 cup or more broth (as above) with crispy fresh vegetables
>   grated in

Day 6

BREAKFAST
Simmer:
> ¼ pound sweetbreads, sliced thin
> Few slices leek

in:
> ½ cup chicken stock prepared from Bone Stock recipe

Add at last minute:
> Few sprigs parsley, cut up

LUNCH
Preheat in wok or heavy skillet:
> 1 teaspoon dark sesame oil

Add and stir-fry till lightly browned:
> 1 clove garlic, thinly sliced
> 1-inch piece fresh ginger, peeled and thinly sliced

Toss in, one at a time, a total of 2 cups or more:
> Chinese cabbage, shredded
> Bamboo shoots, sliced thin
> Cucumber, sliced thin
> Bean sprouts
> Mushrooms, sliced
> Spinach, coarsely shredded

Stir-fry briefly, till vegetables are crisp-tender. (An alternative way to prepare vegetables would be to steam them over 1 cup broth, then sprinkle with 1 tablespoon sesame seeds.)

DINNER
Combine:
> ¼ pound lobster meat, steamed
> Asparagus (as much as you want), steamed or raw
> 2 cups or more escarole and/or other mixed dark greens, steamed or raw

Drizzle with:
> Low- or No-Calorie Salad Dressing

SNACK
> ½ cantaloupe

Day 7

BREAKFAST
>2 eggs, poached or boiled
>apricots

LUNCH
Sprinkle:
>¼ cup your choice from Nuts and Seeds list
over:
>1 cup yogurt
Accompany with:
>1 glass carrot juice or other vegetable juice

DINNER
In saucepan, braise gently:
>¼ pound beef heart, cubed or sliced
>1 teaspoon butter
Stir in:
>Onions and other vegetables from the High-Potassium
>   Foods list (as much as you want), chopped
Cover with:
>1–2 cups broth from Basic High-Potassium Soup or Bone
>   Stock recipe
Simmer till beef heart is tender and vegetables are done to your liking.

SNACK
>½ grapefruit

Day 8

BREAKFAST
Spoon:
>¼ cup toasted wheat germ
>1 tablespoon oat bran
>1 tablespoon blackstrap molasses
over:
>1 cup yogurt

LUNCH
Serve on half shell:
    6 raw oysters
Accompany with:
    1 cup Brussels sprouts, steamed
seasoned with:
    1 clove garlic
    1 teaspoon dark sesame oil
    1 teaspoon rice vinegar (or other)
Add a salad of:
    2–4 cups dark leafy greens
    Low- or No-Calorie Salad Dressing

DINNER
Sauté:
    ½–1 onion, sliced
till just brown in:
    1 teaspoon butter
Then add:
    ¼ pound liver, thinly sliced
Cook gently till barely done. Serve with:
    1 glass fresh vegetable juice (your choice)

SNACK
    ¼ cantaloupe

Day 9
BREAKFAST
Sprinkle:
    ¼ cup your choice from Nuts and Seeds list
over:
    1 cup yogurt
Serve with:
    ¼ fresh pineapple, cut up

LUNCH
Arrange:
    ¼ pound shrimp, steamed

on a bed of:
>1–2 cups spinach, steamed just till wilted

Top with:
>Low- or No-Calorie Salad Dressing

Accompany with:
>Your choice of raw vegetables from the High-Potassium
>Foods list, cut up as finger food

DINNER
Preheat in wok or heavy skillet:
>1 teaspoon oil

Toss in and stir-fry briefly:
>1 clove garlic, minced
>1-inch piece fresh ginger, thinly sliced

Add and stir-fry until lightly browned:
>¼ pound beef or veal heart, cut into cubes

Toss in and continue stir-frying till just done:
>1 cup shredded cabbage or kale

Serve with:
>Large green salad with alfalfa sprouts
>Low- or No-Calorie Salad Dressing

SNACK
>1 cup pineapple *or* 2 apricots *or* ¼ cantaloupe

Day 10
BREAKFAST
Cook gently together:
>½ pound oysters
>1 teaspoon butter

Then add:
>½ cup warm milk

Heat through and serve.

LUNCH
>½ cup cottage cheese
>½ cantaloupe

DINNER

Cut into small pieces:
   ¼ pound sweetbreads
Dip them in:
   1 beaten egg
then roll in:
   2 tablespoons toasted wheat germ, seasoned
Cook gently in:
   1 teaspoon butter
Serve with:
   3 whole endives, steamed
Add a salad of:
   Butterhead lettuce (use a whole head if you want)
   Low- or No-Calorie Salad Dressing

SNACK
   1 peach or other fruit choice

Nutrient Analysis

These tables show the average daily nutrients supplied by the Shine Diet so you can see how they compare with standard recommendations. Figures include the nutrients provided by the basic diet as listed in the daily menus, and the nutrients supplied if my recommendation to use the High-Nutrient Soup as a supplement is followed. The averages are based on the ten-day total for each nutrient, and the figures have been rounded off. (For a fuller discussion of what the figures mean, turn to page 49.)

The Shine (Anti-Stress) Diet:
Meeting Your Needs for Nutrients Having Established RDA *

	RDA		Daily Average Supplied by Diet	
Nutrient	Woman Aged 23–50	Man Aged 23–50	Basic Diet, No Additions	Total with Soup Addition
Vitamin A	4000 IU	5000 IU	31,475 IU	41,515 IU
Vitamin B-1	1.0 mg	1.4 mg	1.46 mg	2.03 mg
Vitamin B-2	1.2 mg	1.6 mg	3.9 mg	4.9 mg
Vitamin B-3	13 mg	18 mg	19.6 mg	26.4 mg
Vitamin B-6	2.0 mg	2.2 mg	1.84 mg	2.84 mg
Vitamin B-12	3.0 mcg	3.0 mcg	48.4 mcg	52.9 mcg
Vitamin C	60 mg	60 mg	318 mg	538 mg
Calcium	800 mg	800 mg	816 mg	1224 mg
Vitamin D†	200 IU	200 IU	—	—
Vitamin E	11.9 IU	14.9 IU	19.6 IU	25 IU
Folacin	400 mcg	400 mcg	431 mcg	760 mcg
Iodine†	150 mcg	150 mcg	—	—
Iron	18 mg	10 mg	26.9 mg	34.7 mg
Magnesium	300 mg	350 mg	280 mg	485 mg
Phosphorus	800 mg	800 mg	1320 mg	1695 mg
Protein	44 gm	56 gm	78.6 gm	93.9 gm
Zinc	15 mg	15 mg	47 mg	52.3 mg

Nutrient values of daily menus were calculated with Health-Aide nutrition software, Programming Technology Corporation, San Rafael, California, 1982.

* The Recommended Dietary Allowances (RDA) are taken from Committee on Dietary Allowances, Food and Nutrition Board, *Recommended Dietary Allowances* (ninth revised edition), Washington, D.C. Complete information for age groups other than those listed here, and for pregnant or lactating women, may be found on page 291.

† Nutrient values for vitamin D and iodine are indeterminate, but it is very unlikely that anyone will get less than the full RDA daily if milk or fish is included in the diet.

gm = gram   IU = international unit   mcg = microgram   mg = milligram

The Shine (Anti-Stress) Diet: Other Important Nutritional Needs

| Nutrient | Recommendation* | Daily Average Supplied by Diet | | Comment† |
		Basic Diet, No Additions	Total with Soup Addition	
Calories	Varies	908	1153	Add treats or needs or both to bring calories to desired level
Carbohydrates	Approximately 58% total calories	82 gm	132 gm	Carbohydrates = about 48% daily calories
Crude Fiber	6 gm or more	7 gm	13.5 gm	Strain the soup if it has too much roughage for you
Potassium	1875–5625 mg	3486 mg	5807 mg	Stay on the high side
All Fats‡	Not to exceed 30% total calories	33 gm	35.1 gm	⎫
Saturated	Approximately 10% total calories	5 gm	5.1 gm	⎬ Fats = 27% daily calories (4% saturated, 5.7% monounsaturated, 5.5% polyunsaturated)
Monounsaturated	Approximately 10% total calories	7 gm	7.3 gm	
Polyunsaturated	Approximately 10% total calories	7 gm	7 gm	⎭
Cholesterol	300 mg maximum	928 mg	938 mg	Cholesterol intake is 309% recommended maximum! This diet not for persons whose blood cholesterol level exceeds 150–200 mg
Sodium	1100–3300 mg maximum	885 mg	1171 mg	Keep on the low side
Sugar	Not to exceed 10% total calories	5 gm	5 gm	Sugar = 1.7% daily calories

Nutrient values of daily menus were calculated with Health-Aide nutrition software, Programming Technology Corporation, San Rafael, California, 1982.
 * Nutrient Recommendations regarding carbohydrates, fats, cholesterol, and sugar are part of the Dietary Goals for the United States, prepared by the Senate Select Committee on Nutrition and Human Needs, 1977. Other recommendations are broad guidelines as reported in *Recommended Dietary Allowances.*
 † Percentages are based on total with soup addition.
 ‡ Because values are not available for some minor fatty acids, the amounts listed in each group do not add up to the total for all fats.

Customizing the Diet

CALCULATING CALORIE NEEDS
1. Enter here your daily calorie needs or goals: _____
   (Use the table on page 50, or follow the guidelines in
   Chapter 12 for finding your personal balance. Remember, for best health results, women should generally consume no fewer than 1200 calories daily, and
   men no fewer than 1500, for any extended period of
   time.)
2. This is the average daily number of calories in the
   basic diet, without additions: 908
3. Subtract step 2 from step 1 to learn how many additional calories daily you will require, on average: _____

FILLING YOUR NEEDS: SOME SUGGESTIONS
1. As shown in the nutrient analysis tables, adding *half* the High-
   Nutrient Soup recipe (see page 228) *daily* completes nutritional
   requirements while adding just 245 calories per day.
2. If you choose not to use the High-Nutrient Soup, the lists in
   Food Sources of Major Nutrients, Chapter 17, will help you
   select foods to meet your nutritional needs. Women, for example, could forgo the soup and round out nutrient requirements by adding 1 cup watercress or 1 cup raw spinach each
   day. Men could add 1 cup cooked spinach and 1 cup tomato
   juice. (Because of the high cholesterol content, though, men
   with significant cholesterol levels will want to steer clear of this
   diet.)
3. Once you are sure your nutrient needs are taken care of, you
   can add other foods you like to bring your calorie intake to the
   desired level. The lists in Chapter 14 will help you make good
   choices. You may want to choose a few foods to increase carbohydrates slightly.

How Is the Diet Going?

The checklists and chart will help you keep track of how you're feeling and how you're doing on this diet. Paying close attention to your body's signals may help you determine whether this is the diet for you.

The Shine (Anti-Stress) Diet: Daily Checklist of Negative and Positive Factors

	DAY									
NEGATIVE FACTORS	1	2	3	4	5	6	7	8	9	10
Constipated										
Diarrhea										
Sleepless										
Irritable										
Itchy										
Sneezing										
Hungry										
Headache										
Blackout										
Gas										
Heartburn										
Bloat										
Weakness										
Fatigue										
Nervous										
Anxious										
Tremors										

POSITIVE FACTORS

Bowel movement*										
Sleeping well										
Stomach satisfied										
Alert, clear-headed										
Feel strong										
Lively										

* 1–3 times/day with regular, well-formed stool

The Shine (Anti-Stress) Diet: Daily Weight Change Chart

The horizontal line through the middle of the chart represents your starting weight (Day 1). Each day, mark a new point to show how your weight is changing (or not) as the diet progresses. Draw a line from point to point to chart your weight change.

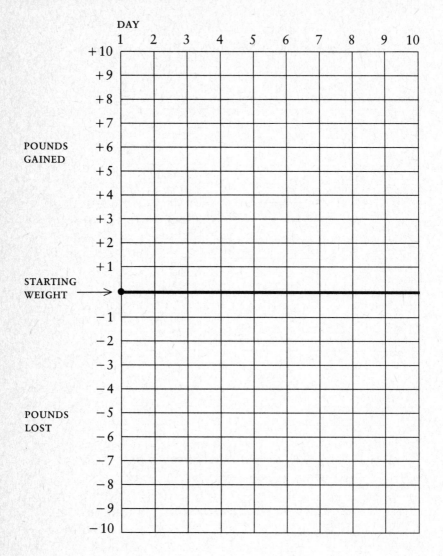

Special Note on Progressive Diseases

People with chronic or progressive diseases — such as diabetes, multiple sclerosis, or arthritis — are often sicker than can be accounted for by the disease itself. Bad nutrition, inactivity, and depression add their effects, often speeding up the decline of health. This accelerated decline can be slowed even though the basic disease process may be of the sort that can't be changed. Very often you can come to a much better condition mentally and physically than would have seemed possible. And that is simply because the process of any disease is magnified by poor diet and inactivity.

A good way of looking at this problem is to take aging itself as a case of a fatal disease. It is obvious by now that many of the weaknesses and debilities that accompany aging are unnecessarily worsened by inadequate nutrition, lack of moving about, and a feeling of hopelessness. Of these, poor eating and simply sitting passively by themselves are enough to account for the hopelessness and the significant speeding up of the natural decline.

If you have a progressive disease that weakens you, it is important to try to build yourself up against the stress of the disease. Since the body absorbs nutrients on an ongoing basis, day by day, hour by hour, minute by minute, eat well and often. When you go about this methodically and stubbornly, never letting a day or a meal or a snack go by without encouraging your body with the right food, you will, in every case that I've seen, begin to build health *in spite of the disease*. Once you have gone through several months of eating well, you will find that your health is continuing to improve and that more and more of the problems that you thought were caused by the disease have begun to recede. You may find that the progressions of the illness that you have are becoming less frequent and less severe. You may find that systems in your body that you thought were lost forever are beginning to work again. You may find that your energy level has lifted, that people are beginning to tell you how good you look, that your doctor is not so unhappy to see you walk through the door. And you will learn that even with a progressive disease there is some control through the use of good nutrition. As you begin to feel better and more capable, you may want to add those physical activities that are best for you.

It was my own gratifying experience with clients over the years that led me to develop the Shine Diet to its present state. It is designed to provide you with a steady stream of concentrated nutrients to allow for better absorption. All of the diets in this book are nutritionally sound, but I believe this diet to be the best for those who have shortchanged themselves nutritionally over the years, whether or not they have a progressive disease, and also for those who are under constant stress.

Be sure to discuss this diet with your doctor before you begin. Your doctor's nutritional strategies come first.

✿ 8 ✿

The Two-Minute Diet

You can drink your nutrients. For ordinary people in a hurry, for someone recovering from an illness, and for the elderly with their varied problems of weakness, osteoporosis, false teeth (or no teeth), lack of saliva or thick and ropy saliva, I have assembled a set of drinks that are pleasant and easy to take in. They are simple to prepare, tasty going down, and nutritious. The Two-Minute Diet calls for eight drinks a day as opposed to three meals a day because in aging, stress, illness, or disease, the less efficient or overworked system needs a boost more often.

Preparing a meal in two minutes is easy. Eating (drinking) a meal in two minutes is easy also and can give you a whole new range of approaches to healthy eating. The Two-Minute Diet is important for many reasons. This diet, like the others in this book, meets all the Recommended Daily Dietary Allowances when supplemented along the lines suggested at the end of this chapter. It also has some very special attributes that make it particularly good for problems that often accompany aging.

Getting Enough Calcium

Females — both women and girls — are least likely to meet the RDA requirements for calcium. Since only three out of ten families do meet these requirements, and since many more men than women eat enough calories to ensure an adequate intake, perhaps 50 percent of women regularly fail to meet the RDA.

Osteoporosis occurs most frequently among women over fifty years of age, though the condition has been found in teenagers. It is characterized by too little bone (or, literally translated, porous bones), and occurs when you cannot supply or absorb calcium and other minerals in the bones faster than they are taken away. It is normal for the minerals in bone to be laid down and taken away on a very steady and regular basis. The supply and absorption of calcium begins to be more difficult as early as age thirty-five. Your job is to see to it that there is always enough calcium in your system to replace what is pulled out. After menopause a changed hormonal balance makes the laying back down of calcium more difficult, if not impossible, especially for women of northern European background. Surveys show that about 30 percent of women over fifty-five and men over sixty have lost enough bone to result in fractures.

One easy way to guess whether you are beginning to suffer bone loss is to measure your height. All the women I have worked with who have osteoporosis have also lost soft tissue and some inches in height. The loss usually starts at about age forty to fifty and proceeds from there. Many women measure a height loss of up to one inch as early as their forties, and I have worked with women in their seventies who are as much as seven inches shorter than they were when younger. The ten years or so immediately before and after the cessation of menstrual flow seem to be the time of greatest change. The systems then begin to slowly stabilize again, though at a lesser level, leaving most women feeling a little more fragile.

You can lose calcium from the jaw, which causes your teeth to loosen, many times resulting in the loss of your teeth. This is important, because dentures do only about a third of the work that your own natural teeth do in chewing.

Calcium loss from the bones of your spine (vertebrae) most often shows up in in symptoms of low back pain, then neck and arm pain, then midback pain, usually in that order in my experience. The first sign for the majority of women is early-morning low backache on a regular basis. This is because most calcium is lost when fasting (the hours between dinner and breakfast) and when your body weight is not on your legs, reminding the body that it needs more minerals in this particular place.

Are you sleeping wrong — do you really need a new mattress — or is your backache really the first sign of osteoporosis? Are you really clenching or grinding your teeth at night, or is it the first sign of osteoporosis? That tingling down your neck and arms and hands and in your toes — is it something else or a symptom of osteoporosis?

And then there are stresses that cause osteoporosis. Trauma, chilling, starvation, dehydration, surgery, and fear — the net effect is osteoporosis and the breaking down of the soft tissues of the spine. Under stress you can actually pull the calcium from your bones and tissues to the point that you are excreting twice as much calcium as you are taking in, even though you are taking in the amount that keeps you in calcium balance when you are *not* under stress. Only the reduction of stress or a much higher intake of calcium will bring the calcium into balance.

How often are you under stress? For how long a period of time? Some stress is normal to life. Does yours fall into the normal range, or is it constant or daily? Right now is a good time to think about the kind of condition you want to be in ten, twenty, thirty, or forty years from now. It takes time, effort, and consistency to recondition your body to habits that will better preserve your health and quality of life. The longer you wait, the fewer of your essential systems will be in good working order, the longer the reconditioning will take, and the less will be achieved.

Eating and Aging

Many of us, as we age, lose the ability to produce the amount of saliva necessary to make swallowing easy. What saliva there is, is often thick and ropy. Its stickiness causes difficulties in chewing, in tasting, in moving the food freely around in the mouth, and in swallowing. It can cause dry food to adhere to the gums and result in irritations, and it often causes us to stop eating properly. The higher the age, generally the worse the problem becomes.

Another problem related to aging is that degenerative changes of the digestive glands may cause gastrointestinal changes without disease occurring. These changes usually begin at around age fifty.

Because of the loss of teeth, the sticky saliva, and the loss of ease in digestion, many of us as we grow older stop eating meat and vegetables, which require chewing, and especially raw vegetables, which require a little more of our digestive tract. Then we tend to lack protein and potassium and the strength these foods would normally give us. If we continue in this fashion, our bodies will degenerate at an ever-increasing rate.

Forget this horror story! The Two-Minute Diet provides a full complement of highly nutritious foods, cut into such fine particles that your digestive system has no need to do the large job of breaking them down initially, in a fluid base that allows you to swallow them easily and prevents their sticking to your gums and palate. Eating (drinking) can become a pleasure again. Meat, vegetables, dairy products, are all provided in a form that requires very little work for your hands, such as cleaning and cutting up, or your jaws, such as chewing. You will probably find that you eat more — as you should — because the diet is simple and easy. And you will feel better because you are eating very well and are better able to digest more.

A healthy system, on the other hand, *should* be put to the test. If you don't need this diet, don't bother unless you're in such a hurry you might go without eating well unless the preparation is made quick and easy. But if you feel too tired to eat, too lonely to eat, have too little time to eat, have dentures that make it too troublesome to eat, be smart. You may choose not to follow the diet plan in its entirety, but you can still add just a couple of these drinks to improve your regular diet of fresh foods; or during the day have five of these drinks and then eat your regular dinner. Use your imagination. Make the drinks taste even better. Add any herbs or spices you like. Heat up the drinks or make them icy cold. Get yourself a blender and live happily and healthily with the help of the Two-Minute Diet. It may literally be a lifesaver!

Shopping List

A bullet (•) indicates the specific foods called for in the daily menus. The other listed foods would be good additions to the core diet. To make sure canned and bottled foods have no added sugar or salt — *read labels!*

SEAFOOD (canned)
- mackerel (bone in)
- oysters
- salmon (bone in)
  sardines (bone in)
- shrimp

MEATS
- liver paste

DAIRY PRODUCTS (all lowfat, no added salt or sugar; cultured if available)
- buttermilk
  cheeses
  - cottage cheese
    farmer cheese
  - ricotta cheese
  eggs
  laban (thickened yogurt)
- milk

- powdered milk
  sweet acidophilus milk
- yogurt

VEGETABLES AND VEGETABLE JUICES (no added salt)
- tomato juice
- tomato paste
- V-8 juice

FRUITS AND FRUIT JUICES (no added sugar)
- apricot nectar
  apricots
- currants, dried
- peaches
- peach nectar
- pear nectar
  prune juice
- prunes, dried

NUTS, SEEDS, AND GRAINS (unroasted, unsalted)
  almonds
  Brazil nuts
  oat bran
- peanut butter
  pecans
  pumpkin seeds
  sesame seeds
  sunflower seeds
  walnuts
- wheat germ (toasted)
- wheat bran (fine)

OTHER
- blackstrap molasses
- chives or scallions
- curry powder
- dill
- tofu

Daily Menus

Mix, blend, or whip together the separate drinks listed for each day. Serve hot, cold, or frozen. You may prefer to eat some of the mixes, such as those with cottage cheese, as a soft meal. Drink (or eat) them at whatever time you choose.

Have These Five Drinks Daily

    6 ounces milk
    1 tablespoon blackstrap molasses

6 ounces apricot nectar
1 tablespoon toasted wheat germ

6 ounces milk
2 tablespoons fine wheat or oat bran

6 ounces V-8 or tomato juice
2 tablespoons tofu

6 ounces apricot nectar
1 tablespoon yogurt

Have These in Addition to the Five Daily Drinks
Day 1
6 ounces milk
2 ounces pear nectar

6 ounces milk
2 teaspoons peanut butter

6 ounces milk
2 tablespoons tomato paste

Day 2
6 ounces milk
2 ounces canned liver paste

6 ounces milk
1 heaping teaspoon nuts or seeds

6 ounces milk or cottage cheese
3½ ounces canned, drained shrimp

Day 3
6 ounces milk
¼ cup canned oysters

6 ounces apricot nectar
2 tablespoons cottage cheese

6 ounces milk
1 heaping tablespoon nuts and seeds

Day 4
　　6 ounces peach nectar
　　1 tablespoon ricotta cheese

　　6 ounces buttermilk
　　2 ounces V-8 juice

　　6 ounces yogurt
　　2 dried, soaked, pitted prunes

Day 5
　　6 ounces yogurt
　　1 heaping teaspoon nuts and seeds

　　6 ounces milk
　　1 tablespoon dried, soaked currants

　　6 ounces yogurt
　　2 tablespoons canned salmon

Day 6
　　6 ounces milk
　　peach half, cut up

　　6 ounces yogurt or cottage cheese
　　½ can shrimp
　　Dill or curry to taste

　　6 ounces V-8 juice
　　1 tablespoon powdered milk

Day 7
　　6 ounces yogurt
　　2 dried, soaked, pitted prunes

　　6 ounces apricot nectar
　　2 tablespoons yogurt

　　6 ounces milk
　　2 tablespoons tomato paste

Day 8
>   6 ounces milk
>   2 ounces canned liver paste
>
>   6 ounces apricot nectar
>   1 tablespoon ricotta cheese
>
>   6 ounces cottage cheese
>   3½ ounces canned, drained shrimp
>   Scallions or chives cut up into mix
>   Dill or curry to taste

Day 9
>   6 ounces buttermilk
>   2 ounces peach nectar
>
>   6 ounces cottage or ricotta cheese
>   1 tablespoon canned mackerel
>
>   6 ounces yogurt
>   1 tablespoon nuts and seeds

Day 10
>   6 ounces milk
>   2 teaspoons smooth peanut butter
>
>   6 ounces cottage or ricotta cheese
>   2 tablespoons canned salmon
>   1–2 teaspoons chopped scallion (if desired)
>
>   6 ounces peach nectar
>   1 tablespoon powdered milk

Nutrient Analysis

These tables show the average daily nutrients supplied by the Two-Minute Diet so you can see how they compare with standard recommendations. Figures include the nutrients provided by the basic diet as listed in the daily menus, and the nutrients supplied if my recommendation to use the High-Nutrient Soup as a supplement is followed. The averages are based on the ten-day total for each nutrient, and the figures have been rounded off. (For a fuller discussion of what the figures mean, turn to page 49.)

The Two-Minute Diet: Meeting Your Needs for Nutrients Having Established RDA *

	RDA		Daily Average Supplied by Diet	
Nutrient	Woman Aged 23–50	Man Aged 23–50	Basic Diet, No Additions	Total with Soup Addition
Vitamin A	4000 IU	5000 IU	10,350 IU	20,390 IU
Vitamin B-1	1.0 mg	1.4 mg	0.82 mg	1.4 mg
Vitamin B-2	1.2 mg	1.6 mg	2.16 mg	3.16 mg
Vitamin B-3	13 mg	18 mg	11.2 mg	18 mg
Vitamin B-6	2.0 mg	2.2 mg	1.1 mg	2.1 mg
Vitamin B-12	3.0 mcg	3.0 mcg	15 mcg	19.5 mcg
Vitamin C	60 mg	60 mg	54.6 mg	275 mg
Calcium	800 mg	800 mg	1520 mg	1928 mg
Vitamin D †	200 IU	200 IU	—	—
Vitamin E	11.9 IU	14.9 IU	8.9 IU	14.3 IU
Folacin	400 mcg	400 mcg	188 mcg	517 mcg
Iodine †	150 mcg	150 mcg	—	—
Iron	18 mg	10 mg	14.8 mg	22.6 mg
Magnesium	300 mg	350 mg	387 mg	592 mg
Phosphorus	800 mg	800 mg	1480 mg	1855 mg
Protein	44 gm	56 gm	58.5 gm	73.8 gm
Zinc	15 mg	15 mg	11.7 mg	17 mg

Nutrient values of daily menus were calculated with Health-Aide nutrition software, Programming Technology Corporation, San Rafael, California, 1982.

* The Recommended Dietary Allowances (RDA) are taken from Committee on Dietary Allowances, Food and Nutrition Board, *Recommended Dietary Allowances* (ninth revised edition), Washington, D.C. Complete information for age groups other than those listed here, and for pregnant or lactating women, may be found on page 291.

† Nutrient values for vitamin D and iodine are indeterminate, but it is very unlikely that anyone will get less than the full RDA daily if milk or fish is included in the diet.

gm = gram   IU = international unit   mcg = microgram   mg = milligram

The Two-Minute Diet: Other Important Nutritional Needs

Nutrient	Recommendation *	Daily Average Supplied by Diet		Comment †
		Basic Diet, No Additions	Total with Soup Addition	
Calories	Varies	1080	1325	Add treats or needs or both to bring calories to desired level
Carbohydrates	Approximately 58% total calories	150 gm	200 gm	Carbohydrates = about 60% daily calories
Crude Fiber	6 gm or more	3 gm	9.5 gm	
Potassium	1875–5625 mg	3818 mg	6139 mg	Stay on the high side
All Fats ‡	Not to exceed 30% total calories	29 gm	31.1 gm	
Saturated	Approximately 10% total calories	14 gm	14.1 gm	Fats = 21% daily calories (10% saturated, 5.6% monounsaturated, 2% polyunsaturated)
Monounsaturated	Approximately 10% total calories	8 gm	8.3 gm	
Polyunsaturated	Approximately 10% total calories	3 gm	3 gm	
Cholesterol	300 mg maximum	97 mg	107 mg	Keep on the low side
Sodium	1100–3300 mg maximum	1079 mg	1365 mg	Keep on the low side
Sugar	Not to exceed 10% total calories	18 gm	18 gm	Sugar = 5.5% daily calories

Nutrient values of daily menus were calculated with Health-Aide nutrition software, Programming Technology Corporation, San Rafael, California, 1982.

 * Nutrient Recommendations regarding carbohydrates, fats, cholesterol, and sugar are part of the Dietary Goals for the United States, prepared by the Senate Select Committee on Nutrition and Human Needs, 1977. Other recommendations are broad guidelines as reported in *Recommended Dietary Allowances.*

 † Percentages are based on total with soup addition.

 ‡ Because values are not available for some minor fatty acids, the amounts listed in each group do not add up to the total for all fats.

Customizing the Diet

CALCULATING CALORIE NEEDS
1. Enter here your daily calorie needs or goals: _____
   (Use the table on page 50, or follow the guidelines in Chapter 12 for finding your personal balance. Remember, for best health results, women should generally consume no fewer than 1200 calories daily, and men no fewer than 1500, for any extended period of time.)
2. This is the average daily number of calories in the basic diet, without additions: 1080
3. Subtract step 2 from step 1 to learn how many additional calories daily you will require, on average: _____

FILLING YOUR NEEDS: SOME SUGGESTIONS
1. As shown in the nutrient analysis tables, adding *half* the High-Nutrient Soup recipe (see page 228) *daily* completes most nutritional requirements while adding just 245 calories per day. If you choose not to use the High-Nutrient Soup, the lists in Food Sources of Major Nutrients, Chapter 17, will help you select foods to meet your nutritional needs. You could, for example, forgo the soup and instead add these foods daily (blenderized if you want a fully liquid diet):

   1 cup asparagus
   2 small bananas or other B-6 food
   ½ cup strawberries
   4 ounces beef liver or other folacin source
   1 oyster or other zinc source

   Women will need to add another iron source daily, such as 1 cup cooked spinach, to meet the RDA.
   To meet vitamin B-1 and B-3 requirements, men should also add 1 cup peas and 1 cup mushrooms, or the equivalent, daily.
2. Even with the soup addition, men will need to make sure they get enough vitamins B-6 and E. Adding the asparagus daily would cover these requirements.
3. Once you are sure your nutrient needs are taken care of, add other foods you like to bring your calorie intake to the desired level. The lists in Chapter 14 will help you make good choices.

How Is the Diet Going?
The checklists and chart will help you keep track of how you're feeling and how you're doing on this diet. Paying close attention to your body's signals may help you determine whether this is the diet for you.

The Two-Minute Diet:
Daily Checklist of Negative and Positive Factors

NEGATIVE FACTORS	DAY 1	2	3	4	5	6	7	8	9	10
Constipated										
Diarrhea										
Sleepless										
Irritable										
Itchy										
Sneezing										
Hungry										
Headache										
Blackout										
Gas										
Heartburn										
Bloat										
Weakness										
Fatigue										
Nervous										
Anxious										
Tremors										

POSITIVE FACTORS

Bowel movement*										
Sleeping well										
Stomach satisfied										
Alert, clear-headed										
Feel strong										
Lively										

* 1–3 times/day with regular, well-formed stool

The Two-Minute Diet: Daily Weight Change Chart

The horizontal line through the middle of the chart represents your starting weight (Day 1). Each day, mark a new point to show how your weight is changing (or not) as the diet progresses. Draw a line from point to point to chart your weight change.

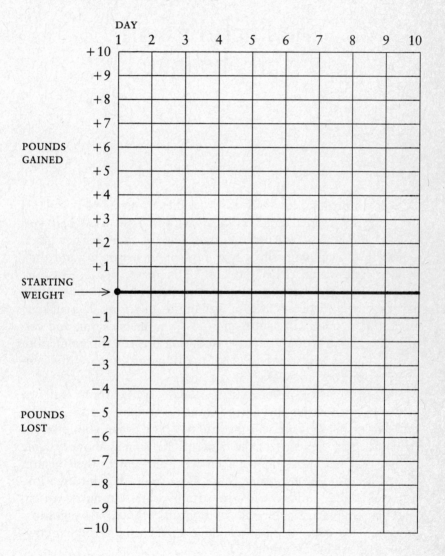

❧ 9 ❧

The High-Protein,
Low-Carbohydrate Diet

The high-protein, low-carbohydrate diet that was so popular a few years ago carried some problems with it. True, it did help you to lose weight — if you were a man. For the most part, women would lose weight up till a few days premenstrually, and then their weight would either level off or increase. Because of hormonal differences between men and women, this is usually not a diet that helps women to lose weight steadily, nor does it keep them feeling good. The shifts in potassium, magnesium, and calcium levels that women experience during their menstrual period, and the inability of some to catch up afterward, makes this generally a poor diet for women.

The high level of protein and the low level of carbohydrates in early versions of this diet were meant to produce ketosis, which shifts your metabolism, causing you to break down your store of body fats. But the levels of the minerals mentioned above became so low that many people lost their hair, along with their health. This is not a necessary result. With more up-to-date information, we can include foods very low in carbohydrates but nutrient-rich, which will replace the minerals without disturbing the weight-loss process. This is what has been done in the High-Protein, Low-Carbohydrate Diet, outlined below.

Ketosis is a natural process of the body, which sees us through emergency periods when food is not available. Fasting will also kick us into ketosis. Many zoos fast their animals at least one day a week just to keep this natural ability in working order. Obviously, though it is an ability we need to have available to us, ketosis is still an emergency measure. Emergencies are stressful. Some stress is good and keeps you on your toes. Too much is too much. Ketosis brings shakiness and blackouts to some people. If you feel good on this diet, fine! If not—quit!

The High-Protein, Low-Carbohydrate Diet would probably be a good weight-loss diet for men, though no more than one ten-day period a year. Otherwise, maintain yourself, or lose weight, on a more stabilizing diet.

Problems with the High-Protein, Low-Carbohydrate Diet

The High-Protein, Low-Carbohydrate Diet is the only one in this book that I consider to be just barely acceptable, even though it differs in a number of important ways from most diets of this type. I have revised it particularly to increase greatly the electrolytes — potassium, calcium, and magnesium — in which many versions of this diet are too low. This type of diet can also be extremely low in roughage. When protein is used by the digestive system it leaves very little residue. This causes great straining in passing the residue through the digestive tract and results in a very small stool, often accompanied by much discomfort. I have added as much roughage as I could without disturbing too greatly the low-carbohydrate aspect of the diet.

You should be aware that in general high-protein diets are nutritionally unbalanced and often they are ineffective, as weight lost is often regained. Possible side effects include fatigue, apathy, and nausea. Such a diet is dangerous for persons with heart disease, gout, kidney disease, diabetes, persons on certain medication, and pregnant women. Play it safe and check with your physician before embarking on this or any other version of a high-protein diet.

Another point. It is common sense in this day and age to know what your blood cholesterol level is. This diet, because it is high in protein from flesh, is ordinarily high in cholesterol also. *It doesn't have to be!* You can easily arrange to have one, two, or even three meals a day consist of fatty fish rather than beef, lamb, or pork. (Some of the fatty fish are bluefish, mackerel, tuna, sardines, shad, butterfish, and salmon.) The fish are high in long-chain fatty acids that lower triglyceride and cholesterol levels in your blood. If that seems too troublesome to you, try taking a daily swallow of cod-liver oil (2000 international units vitamin A, 200 international units vitamin D), which also contains generous amounts of these fatty acids. Be sure to buy a reputable brand that comes sealed. Once it has been opened, be sure to keep the oil in the refrigerator. All oils become rancid very quickly when not kept cold. Buying smaller containers helps to keep your supply fresh. (The names of the long-chain fatty acids mentioned above for those of you who might want to investigate further are eicosapentaenoic acid, EPA, and docosahexaenoic acid, DHA. Not of the least importance if you don't want to know.)

Important Notes on the High-Protein, Low-Carbohydrate Diet

The reason for the large number of vegetables and fruits in this diet is to prevent a loss of potassium, magnesium, and calcium. These important minerals and possibly others are lost quickly on a high-protein diet and must be replaced immediately. Do not neglect to keep up your intake of the suggested vegetables and fruits.

Under ordinary circumstances you could expect to have fewer and smaller bowel movements on a high-protein diet since fiber content would be on the low side and because high-protein foods leave very little bulk. We have increased the low-carbohydrate vegetable intake to try to prevent this problem.

A diet high in animal flesh is also going to be generally high in fat. Remember that there are always some hidden fats in the leanest meats and chicken. *If you can see fat on it, don't buy it!* And keep added fats to a minimum. Use no more than one added teaspoon of fats and one teaspoon of oils daily. There are 35 calories per teaspoon, or 70 added calories a day in the two teaspoons. Acceptable oils and fats in extremely small amounts are:

    olive oil
    sesame oil, light or dark
    linseed oil (only from food stores)
    safflower oil
    corn oil
    butter
    soft margarine

All fats and oils should be bought in the smallest possible containers and kept refrigerated after opening. Rancid fats and oils are as destructive as the fresh ones are constructive.

Shopping List

A bullet (•) indicates the specific foods called for in the daily menus. The other listed foods would be good additions to the core diet.

SEAFOOD (no shellfish)
• bass
• flounder
• haddock
• halibut
• mackerel
  perch (ocean)
• pollock
  scrod
• snapper
• tuna

MEATS (very lean, no organ meats)
• beef
• hamburger
• roast
• sirloin tips
• T-bone steak
  lamb
  veal

POULTRY (young birds, skin removed)
• chicken
• guinea fowl
• turkey

VEGETABLES
• asparagus
  cabbage (red, white, Savoy)
• celery
• chicory
• Chinese cabbage
• cucumbers
• endive
• garlic
• lettuce, looseleaf (all varieties)
• lettuce, romaine
• mushrooms
  okra
• onions
  parsley
• peppers, sweet green and red
• radishes
• scallions
• spinach
• watercress
• zucchini

FRUITS
• cantaloupe
• grapefruit
• honeydew melon
• lemons
• limes
• strawberries
• watermelon

OILS AND FATS (in order of preference)
• olive oil
• dark sesame oil
• butter

OTHER
• fresh ginger
• herbs and spices (celery seed, curry powder, dill weed, marjoram, rosemary)
• tofu (firm)
• vinegar

Daily menus

The basic recipes and food lists referred to in the menus may be found in Chapter 14.

Day 1

BREAKFAST
  ¼ pound T-bone steak (meat only), broiled
  1 cup strawberries

LUNCH
Bake at 200° F for about 20 minutes:
    ½ pound mackerel
Serve with a salad of:
    1–2 cups spinach leaves
    1 cup sliced mushrooms
    No-Calorie Salad Dressing

DINNER
Preheat in wok or heavy skillet:
    1 teaspoon olive oil
Toss in and stir-fry briefly:
    2 cups shredded zucchini
Serve with:
    ½ pound turkey, baked

SNACK
Simmer together until vegetables are tender:
    1 cup turkey broth prepared from Bone Stock recipe
    1 cup chopped vegetables from the Low-Carbohydrate
       Foods list

Day 2
BREAKFAST
Poach:
    ½ pound flounder
in:
    1 cup broth from Basic High-Potassium Soup
    1 clove minced garlic
    Other spices to taste

LUNCH
Broil:
    ¼ pound leanest hamburger
Serve with:
    Onions
    Lettuce
    Radishes

DINNER
Reheat until simmering steadily:
> 1 quart Basic High-Potassium Soup made with Bone Stock
> that has been chilled so all fat can be removed

Just before serving, add:
> ½ pound chicken, slivered and browned gently in 1
> teaspoon olive oil

Then add:
> Rosemary, marjoram, or seasonings you'd like

Save half the soup for tomorrow's breakfast.

SNACK
> ½ grapefruit

Day 3
BREAKFAST
> Chicken soup left over from night before

LUNCH
Prepare either:
> ½ pound sashimi (raw, very fresh fish)

or:
> ½ pound tuna, gently baked at 200° F for 20 minutes

Serve with a salad of:
> Cucumber slices and dill weed (as much as you want)

sprinkled with:
> Vinegar
> Minced garlic

DINNER
Brown:
> ¼ pound beef, cubed
> 1 clove garlic, minced

in:
> 1 teaspoon butter

Stir into:
> 1 pint Bone Stock

along with:
> 1 cup mushrooms, sliced (whole if small)
> Any other vegetables you like from the High-Potassium or
>   Low-Carbohydrate lists, cut up

Simmer until vegetables have the texture you like.

SNACK
> 1 cup strawberries

Day 4

BREAKFAST
Prepare:
> ½ pound haddock

in either of the following ways:
> bake (without added oil) at 200° F for 15–20 minutes
> or *poach in 2 cups broth from Basic High-Potassium Soup*

LUNCH
Toss together:
> ½ pound cooked turkey, sliced or cubed
> Salad greens (looseleaf lettuce, endive, chicory, romaine)
> Low- or No-Calorie Salad Dressing

DINNER
Prepare either:
> ¼ pound leanest hamburger, broiled

or:
> ½ pound fish, your choice, baked

Place on bed of:
> 1–2 cups spinach, wilted (steam 3 minutes or less), and
>   seasoned with 1–2 cloves minced garlic

SNACK
> ¼ cantaloupe *or* ⅛ honeydew melon

Day 5
BREAKFAST
Poach:
>½ pound bass or pollock

in:
>1 cup broth from Basic High-Potassium Soup

Serve on a bed of:
>1 cucumber, sliced
>Dill
>Celery or celery seed

LUNCH
Mix together:
>¼ pound leanest hamburger
>¼ green pepper, chopped
>¼ small onion, chopped

Broil.

DINNER
Season:
>¼ pound chicken

with:
>Curry powder to taste

Bake at 200° F for 20–30 minutes. Serve on a bed of:
>Watercress, fresh or wilted, dressed with No-Calorie Salad
>Dressing

SNACK
>1–4 cups Basic High-Potassium Soup broth

Day 6
BREAKFAST
Prepare either:
>¼ pound sirloin tips, sautéed in 1 teaspoon olive oil

or:
>½ pound fish, your choice, baked at 200° F till done

Season with:
>1 small onion, thinly sliced

LUNCH
Bake at 200° F till done:
    ½ pound halibut
Serve with:
    1 cup mushrooms cooked in 1 cup or less Basic High-
        Potassium Soup broth

DINNER
Roast, or split and broil (no added fat):
    1 guinea fowl
Meanwhile, preheat in wok or heavy skillet:
    1 teaspoon dark sesame oil
Add and stir-fry till lightly browned:
    1 clove garlic, minced
    1-inch piece fresh ginger, cut into matchsticks
Toss in and stir-fry till crisp-tender:
    Cucumbers, sliced
    Chinese cabbage, shredded
    Sweet green pepper, sliced thin
*Serve the vegetables with half the roast guinea fowl (save the
    other half plus some of the vegetables for tomorrow's
    breakfast).*

SNACK
    ¼ cantaloupe, put through blender then placed in freezer till
        almost solid

Day 7
BREAKFAST
    ½ guinea fowl, left over from last night
    Leftover stir-fried vegetables

LUNCH
    3½–4 ounce can water-packed tuna, drained
    10–15 leaves looseleaf lettuce
    1 scallion
    No-Calorie Salad Dressing

DINNER
Either:
 ¼ pound roast beef
or:
 ½ pound fish, baked at 200° F till done
Serve with:
 1–3 cups spinach
wilted in:
 ¼ cup Basic High-Potassium Soup broth, seasoned with
  minced garlic if desired

SNACK
 ⅛ honeydew melon

Day 8
BREAKFAST
Toss together:
 ½ cup cooked turkey, cubed
 4 ounces firm tofu, cubed
 No-Calorie Salad Dressing
 1 scallion, finely chopped

LUNCH
Either:
 ¼ pound steak, broiled
or:
 ½ pound any fish, baked at 200° F till done
Serve with:
 1–4 cups green salad
 No-Calorie Salad Dressing

DINNER
Slice thin and set aside:
 ½ pound snapper
Heat to a steady simmer in a shallow pan:
 2–4 cups Basic High-Potassium Soup (leave vegetables in the
  broth)
*Place snapper in hot soup just before serving (or even in soup
 bowls at the table), as it will cook almost immediately.*

SNACK
>1 cup watermelon balls, *or* 1 small wedge watermelon

Day 9
BREAKFAST
Sauté together:
>¼ pound leanest hamburger meat, in chunks
>1 small onion, sliced
>1 sweet green or red pepper, thinly sliced

LUNCH
Bake at 200° F till done:
>½ pound fish, your choice

Cover with:
>Fresh dill or chives, chopped
>Lemon or lime slices or wedges (or squeeze some over fish)

Serve with a salad of:
>1–3 cups looseleaf lettuce
>No-Calorie Salad Dressing

DINNER
Preheat in wok or heavy skillet:
>1 teaspoon dark sesame oil or olive oil

Toss in and stir-fry:
>¼ pound chicken, cubed
>1 sweet red or green pepper, sliced
>¼ Chinese cabbage, sliced
>2 ounces firm tofu, cubed

Add at last minute, if desired:
>1–2 cups Basic High-Potassium Soup broth

Heat through.

SNACK
>1 cup strawberries

Day 10
BREAKFAST
Preheat in small skillet:
   1 teaspoon olive oil
Add and sauté together:
   ¼ pound leanest hamburger meat
   1 garlic clove, minced
   ½ sweet red pepper, sliced thin
   Curry powder to taste

LUNCH
Bake or poach in broth:
   ½ pound cod
Serve with:
   8 asparagus spears, steamed
   Lemon juice

DINNER
Broil:
   ¼ pound chicken
Serve with a salad of:
   1–3 cups romaine and other looseleaf lettuce
   No-Calorie Dressing

SNACK
   ½ grapefruit

Nutrient Analysis

These tables show the average daily nutrients supplied by the High-Protein, Low-Carbohydrate Diet so you can see how they compare with standard recommendations. Figures include the nutrients provided by the basic diet as listed in the daily menus, and the nutrients supplied if my recommendation to use the High-Nutrient Soup as a supplement is followed. The averages are based on the ten-day total for each nutrient, and the figures have been rounded off. (For a fuller discussion of what the figures mean, turn to page 49.)

The High-Protein, Low-Carbohydrate Diet: Meeting Your Needs for Nutrients Having Established RDA *

	RDA		Daily Average Supplied by Diet	
Nutrient	Woman Aged 23–50	Man Aged 23–50	Basic Diet, No Additions	Total with Soup Addition
Vitamin A	4000 IU	5000 IU	10,550 IU	20,590 IU
Vitamin B-1	1.0 mg	1.4 mg	0.9 mg	1.5 mg
Vitamin B-2	1.2 mg	1.6 mg	1.38 mg	2.4 mg
Vitamin B-3	13 mg	18 mg	30.4 mg	37.2 mg
Vitamin B-6	2.0 mg	2.2 mg	2.5 mg	3.5 mg
Vitamin B-12	3.0 mcg	3.0 mcg	6.1 mcg	10.6 mcg
Vitamin C	60 mg	60 mg	249 mg	469 mg
Calcium	800 mg	800 mg	384 mg	792 mg
Vitamin D†	200 IU	200 IU	—	—
Vitamin E	11.9 IU	14.9 IU	5.4 IU	10.8 IU
Folacin	400 mcg	400 mcg	256 mcg	585 mcg
Iodine†	150 mcg	150 mcg	—	—
Iron	18 mg	10 mg	15.7 mg	23.5 mg
Magnesium	300 mg	350 mg	213 mg	418 mg
Phosphorus	800 mg	800 mg	1300 mg	1675 mg
Protein	44 gm	56 gm	133 gm	148.3 gm
Zinc	15 mg	15 mg	9.5 mg	14.8 mg

Nutrient values of daily menus were calculated with Health-Aide nutrition software, Programming Technology Corporation, San Rafael, California, 1982.

* The Recommended Dietary Allowances (RDA) are taken from Committee on Dietary Allowances, Food and Nutrition Board, *Recommended Dietary Allowances* (ninth revised edition), Washington, D.C. Complete information for age groups other than those listed here, and for pregnant or lactating women, may be found on page 291.

† Nutrient values for vitamin D and iodine are indeterminate, but it is very unlikely that anyone will get less than the full RDA daily if milk or fish is included in the diet.

gm = gram   IU = international unit   mcg = microgram   mg = milligram

The High-Protein, Low-Carbohydrate Diet: Other Important Nutritional Needs

Nutrient	Recommendation*	Daily Average Supplied by Diet		Comment†
		Basic Diet, No Additions	Total with Soup Addition	
Calories	Varies	1208	1453	
Carbohydrates	Approximately 58% total calories	41 gm	91 gm	Carbohydrates = about 25% daily calories; be aware that this type of diet by nature is too low in carbohydrates to be healthful for any length of time
Crude Fiber	6 gm or more	6 gm	12.5 gm	Strain the soup if it has too much roughage for you
Potassium	1875–5625 mg	3412 mg	5733 mg	Stay on the high side
All Fats‡	Not to exceed 30% total calories	53 gm	55.1 gm	Fats = 34% daily calories (9% saturated, 12% monounsaturated, 3% polyunsaturated); you can reduce fats to lower levels by using fish in place of meats
Saturated	Approximately 10% total calories	15 gm	15.1 gm	
Monounsaturated	Approximately 10% total calories	19 gm	19.3 gm	
Polyunsaturated	Approximately 10% total calories	5 gm	5 gm	
Cholesterol	300 mg maximum	277 mg	287 mg	Keep on the low side
Sodium	1100–3300 mg maximum	518 mg	804 mg	Keep on the low side
Sugar	Not to exceed 10% total calories	0 gm	0 gm	

Nutrient values of daily menus were calculated with Health-Aide nutrition software, Programming Technology Corporation, San Rafael, California, 1982.

* Nutrient Recommendations regarding carbohydrates, fats, cholesterol, and sugar are part of the Dietary Goals for the United States, prepared by the Senate Select Committee on Nutrition and Human Needs, 1977. Other recommendations are broad guidelines as reported in *Recommended Dietary Allowances*.

† Percentages are based on total with soup addition.

‡ Because values are not available for some minor fatty acids, the amounts listed in each group do not add up to the total for all fats.

Customizing the Diet

CALCULATING CALORIE NEEDS

1. Enter here your daily calorie needs or goals: _____
   (Use the table on page 50, or follow the guidelines in Chapter 12 for finding your personal balance. Remember, for best health results, men should generally not consume fewer than 1500 calories daily for any extended period of time; this diet is not recommended for women.)

2. This is the average daily number of calories in the   1208
   basic diet, without additions:

3. Subtract step 2 from step 1 to learn how many addi-   _____
   tional calories daily you will require, on average:

FILLING YOUR NEEDS: SOME SUGGESTIONS

1. As shown in the nutrient analysis tables, adding *half* the High-Nutrient Soup recipe (see page 228) *daily* completes most nutritional requirements while adding just 245 calories per day. If you choose not to use the High-Nutrient Soup, the lists in Food Sources of Major Nutrients, Chapter 17, will help you select foods to meet your nutritional needs. Men could, for example, forgo the soup and instead add these foods to the daily diet:

   1 cup asparagus
   1 cup mushrooms
   ½ pound kale
   3 cups raw spinach

2. Even with the soup addition, men will need to keep an eye on vitamin E and zinc levels. Adding 1 cup asparagus along with the soup would take care of this.

3. Once you are sure your nutrient needs are taken care of, you can add other foods you like to bring your calorie intake to the desired level. The lists in Chapter 14 will help you make good choices. If you are determined to maintain the low carbohydrate balance, see especially the list of Low-Carbohydrate Foods.

4. The saturated fat content of the High-Protein, Low-Carbohydrate Diet can be reduced to almost none at all by a shift away

from meats and even poultry. You can choose a variety of ocean fish to keep saturated fats at a minimum. Choose these fish for *no* saturated fats:

abalone	smelt
bluefish	swordfish
shad	tuna, fresh and canned (water-packed)

Choose these fish for *very low* saturated fats (less than 1 gram in ½ pound):

cod	perch (ocean)
flounder	pollock
haddock	snapper
halibut	

How Is the Diet Going?

The checklists and chart will help you keep track of how you're feeling and how you're doing on this diet. Paying close attention to your body's signals may help you determine whether this is the diet for you.

The High-Protein, Low-Carbohydrate Diet: Daily Checklist of Negative and Positive Factors

	DAY									
NEGATIVE FACTORS	1	2	3	4	5	6	7	8	9	10
Constipated										
Diarrhea										
Sleepless										
Irritable										
Itchy										
Sneezing										
Hungry										
Headache										
Blackout										
Gas										
Heartburn										
Bloat										
Weakness										
Fatigue										
Nervous										
Anxious										
Tremors										

POSITIVE FACTORS

Bowel movement*										
Sleeping well										
Stomach satisfied										
Alert, clear-headed										
Feel strong										
Lively										

* 1–3 times/day with regular, well-formed stool

The High-Protein, Low-Carbohydrate Diet:
Daily Weight Change Chart

The horizontal line through the middle of the chart represents your starting weight (Day 1). Each day, mark a new point to show how your weight is changing (or not) as the diet progresses. Draw a line from point to point to chart your weight change.

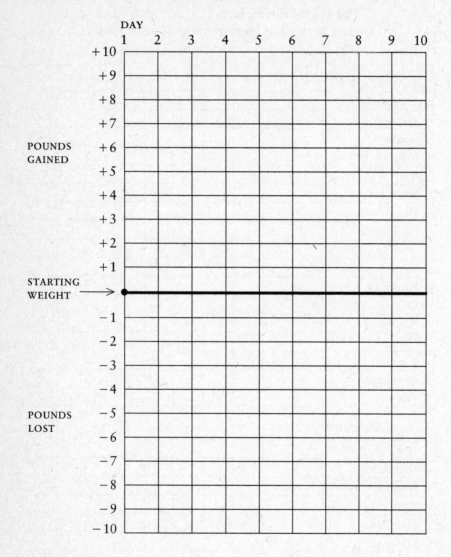

❧ 10 ❧

The Pocket Diet

For the person who is always on the go and has to eat on the run, and for a great many people, such as students and travelers, who don't want leisurely dining but do want to stay healthy, here is a diet based on foods that can be had from the nearest sources, whether it be the corner grocery store or a pantry. It is a diet you can carry around in your pocket (well, maybe a day pack), a diet that can buffer you against your own follies.

Fast Food, Not Junk Food

This diet was interesting to put together because most junk foods and fast foods are directed at just this population. The convenience of junk foods is offset by the poor nutrition that is most often associated with them.

If you really do plan to fix these meals on the move, we assume you'll carry about a fork, a spoon, a can/bottle opener, and a knife of the kind that the police will not mistake as a weapon (perhaps a Swiss Army knife).

There are a number of obvious uses for such a diet — when you're traveling, or can't shop, are snowed in, or cut off as you might be on a boat or an island. We assume that no cooking apparatus, and maybe no water, is easily available. This then becomes a perfect diet for storage in case of emergencies such as power failures (minus, of course, the fresh fruits and vegetables and the fresh milk products).

 When you are in a rush or pressured, it becomes extremely important to remain well nourished.

The Pocket Diet is not the best way for you to eat. It is strictly for emergency, as the name implies. But it supplies most of the nutrients you need. Get onto a regimen of fresh foods and whole foods as soon as possible.

Some Notes on Preserved Foods

At a time when transportation of fresh foods was almost impossible, even unheard of beyond a few miles, simple people in isolated cultures found myriad ways of preserving their foods for coming hard times, whether that was a drought, a poor crop, a long trip to be made, or a long winter season. The food was salted, sugared, fermented, dried, preserved in fat, curdled, cooled, smoked, or hung — wild and wonderful inventions of generations of our ancestors that resulted in their living long enough to get us to this generation and this century.

The Pocket Diet is made up almost completely of foods preserved to withstand time and temperature, but tries to avoid foods with added sugar, salt, fat, or smoke, for safety's sake. Although nutritionally sound, the Pocket Diet is no way to live indefinitely. It is hard to find packaged and prepared foods that are *not* overly salted or sugared, or heavy in fats, or smoked or treated with preservatives and other additives, or all of the above.

Despite the known health hazards, some canned goods still come in cans that are unlined or are sealed with lead. Some of these exposed metals dissolve into the food, especially if the food tends to be acid, such as tomatoes, fruits, and juices. As much as possible choose products that are in glass rather than cans, and in dark glass rather than clear, as light destroys some nutrients.

If there is no alternative to foods on the run for a while, the Pocket Diet meets nutritional needs and will keep you reasonably healthy on preserved foods. But to treat yourself better, try to use as much of the Raw Diet as possible in conjunction with this diet. (The Raw Diet is also easy to eat with virtually no preparation and will tend to keep you much healthier, though it doesn't store as well.) Return to freshly prepared foods as quickly as possible.

Shopping List

A bullet (•) indicates the specific foods called for in the daily menus. The other listed foods would be good additions to the core diet. To make sure canned and bottled foods contain no added salt or sugar — *read labels!*

SEAFOOD (canned)
• crabmeat
• lobster
• mackerel
• oysters, smoked
• salmon
• sardines
• shrimp

MEATS
• liver paste

DAIRY PRODUCTS (all lowfat, no added salt or sugar; cultured if available)
buttermilk
cheeses
• cottage cheese
• hard cheese (such as cheddar or Swiss)
Parmesan cheese
• ricotta cheese
laban (thickened yogurt)
• milk or evaporated milk
sweet acidophilus milk
• yogurt

VEGETABLES (fresh whenever possible)
asparagus
• beans, green (canned)
broccoli
• carrots
• celery
• cucumbers
• garlic
• lettuce, looseleaf
• onions
• peppers, sweet green
• scallions
spinach
• tomatoes (canned)

FRUITS (no added sugar, if canned)
• apricots, canned, fresh, dried
cantaloupe
• currants, dried
grapefruit
• peaches, fresh or dried
• pineapple, canned or dried
• prunes, dried
strawberries

JUICES (no added salt or sugar)
• apricot nectar
peach nectar
• pear nectar

• tomato juice
• V-8 juice (or other vegetable juice)

LEGUMES (canned)
• chickpeas
• kidney beans
lima beans
• navy beans
pinto beans
soybeans

NUTS, SEEDS, AND GRAINS (unroasted, unsalted)
• nuts (all varieties)
• oat bran
• seeds (all varieties)
wheat bran (fine)
• wheat germ (toasted)
• whole-grain bread (no fat)
whole-grain crackers (no fat)

OTHER
• herbs and spices (basil, oregano)
• mayonnaise
• mustard, prepared
• olive oil

Daily Menus

The basic recipes and food lists referred to in the menus may be found in Chapter 14. Without a very cold windowsill or refrigerator for storage, opened canned goods must be consumed within two consecutive meals. Buy small cans and shift meals about as you must.

Day 1

BREAKFAST
Mix together:
> 1 cup yogurt
> 4 apricots, fresh or dried, chopped
> ¼ cup your choice from Nuts and Seeds list

LUNCH
> 4-ounce can sardines
> 1 small onion

DINNER
> 4 ounces canned salmon
> 2 raw carrots

SNACK
Mix together:
> 4 ounces apricot nectar
> ½ cup fresh or reconstituted evaporated milk

Day 2

BREAKFAST
Mix with hot water to thicken:
> ¼ cup toasted wheat germ
> 1 tablespoon oat bran
> 1 tablespoon dried currants

LUNCH
Spread:
> 2 ounces liver paste
on:
> 1 slice whole-grain bread
Serve with:
> Scallions

DINNER
Make a fish salad by mixing together:
     ½ cup canned salmon or mackerel
     1 scallion, cut up
     1 rib celery, diced
     1 teaspoon mayonnaise thinned with 1 teaspoon water
Serve wrapped in 1–10 individual lettuce leaves

SNACK
     2 fresh or dried peaches or prunes

Day 3
BREAKFAST
Sprinkle:
     1 tablespoon oat bran
     2–3 prunes, cut up
over:
     1 cup yogurt

LUNCH
Mix together a fish salad using:
     ½ cup canned mackerel
     1 scallion, cut up
     1 rib celery, diced
     1 teaspoon mayonnaise, thinned with 1 teaspoon water
Serve mixture in:
     1–10 lettuce leaves

DINNER
Mix together:
     10-ounce can beans (chickpeas, navy beans, kidney beans,
        etc.)
     1 onion, chopped
     1 teaspoon prepared mustard
     1 clove garlic, mashed or minced
     6-ounce can V-8 (or tomato juice)
Eat hot or cold according to circumstances.

SNACK
     1 cup pear nectar

Day 4
BREAKFAST
⅛ pound cheddar or Swiss cheese, cut up
4 fresh or dried apricot halves *or* 2 fresh or dried peach
    halves

LUNCH
Mix together:
4-ounce can shrimp
½ cup cottage cheese (chive if you like)
Serve on or wrapped in:
Lettuce leaves

DINNER
4-ounce can smoked oysters
1 cup crushed unsweetened canned pineapple *or* 1 small
    package dried pineapple

SNACK
¼ cup your choice from Nuts and Seeds list

Day 5
BREAKFAST
Mix together:
1 cup cottage cheese
½ cup canned apricots (packed in white grape juice)

LUNCH
Make a bean salad by mixing:
1 cup beans (chickpeas, navy beans, kidney beans, etc.)
1 teaspoon olive oil
1 clove garlic, minced
1 scallion, cut up

DINNER
Mix up a tomato soup:
1–2 cups whole peeled tomatoes, with their juice
Basil to taste
Oregano to taste
1 clove garlic, minced

Accompany with lobster salad made with:
    4-ounce can lobster meat
    1 rib celery, finely diced
    Low- or No-Calorie Salad Dressing

SNACK
    1 cup yogurt

Day 6
BREAKFAST
Mix together:
    1 cup yogurt
    ½ cup apricot nectar *or* peach nectar *or* pear nectar

LUNCH
Mix together:
    ¾ cup canned salmon
    Diced cucumber, celery, and scallion (as much as you want)
    ½ teaspoon olive oil
Spread on:
    3–4 whole-grain crackers (containing no fat)

DINNER
Make a bean salad:
    1 cup beans (navy beans, chickpeas, kidney beans, etc.)
    ½ teaspoon olive oil
    1 clove garlic, minced
    1 scallion, cut up
Serve hot or cold as circumstances permit.

SNACK
    1 cup V-8 juice (or any other vegetable juice)

Day 7
BREAKFAST
> 4-ounce can fruit *or* 1 serving from Fresh Fruits list
> ¼ cup your choice from Nuts and Seeds list

LUNCH
> 1 cup plain yogurt
> 1 serving from Fresh Fruits list

DINNER
> ⅛ pound cheddar or Swiss cheese, cut up
> 1 sweet green pepper
> 1 cucumber
> 1 rib celery

SNACK
> 1 serving from Fresh Fruits list

Day 8
BREAKFAST
Mix together:
> ½ cup cottage cheese
> 1 tablespoon fine wheat bran
> 1 teaspoon dried currants

LUNCH
> 1 serving from Fresh Fruits list
> 1 cup yogurt or milk

DINNER
Mix together:
> 1 can crabmeat, drained
> 1 teaspoon mayonnaise mixed with 1 teaspoon water
Accompany with:
> 6–8 ounces vegetable juice

SNACK
Sprinkle:
> ¼ cup toasted wheat germ *or* 1 tablespoon oat bran
over:
> 4-ounce can fruit

Day 9
BREAKFAST
Mix together till smooth:
>6 ounces fruit nectar
>2 tablespoons yogurt

LUNCH
>4-ounce can sardines, drained
>1 or 2 scallions
>Raw vegetables from the High-Potassium Foods list, as much as you want

DINNER
Stir together:
>1 cup canned beans, mixed varieties (green beans, red kidney beans, white kidney or navy beans)
>1 teaspoon olive oil
>1 small white onion, chopped
>Fresh or dried basil, other herbs as you wish

SNACK
>6 ounces pear nectar

Day 10
BREAKFAST
>¼ cup your choice from Nuts and Seeds list
>1 cup yogurt

LUNCH
>1 cup cottage or ricotta cheese, *or* ⅛ pound cheddar or Swiss cheese
>1 serving from Fresh Fruits list

DINNER
Mix together:
>¾ cup canned salmon or mackerel
>Your choice of raw vegetables, chopped
>1 teaspoon mayonnaise thinned with 1 teaspoon water, *or* 1 teaspoon olive oil

SNACK
>1 serving from Fresh Fruits list

Nutrient Analysis

These tables show the average daily nutrients supplied by the Pocket Diet so you can see how they compare with standard recommendations. Figures include the nutrients provided by the basic diet as listed in the daily menus, and the nutrients supplied if my recommendation to use the High-Nutrient Soup as a supplement is followed. The averages are based on the ten-day total for each nutrient, and the figures have been rounded off. (For a fuller discussion of what the figures mean, turn to page 49.)

The Pocket Diet:
Meeting Your Needs for Nutrients Having Established RDA *

	RDA		Daily Average Supplied by Diet	
Nutrient	Woman Aged 23–50	Man Aged 23–50	Basic Diet, No Additions	Total with Soup Addition
Vitamin A	4000 IU	5000 IU	5600 IU	15,640 IU
Vitamin B-1	1.0 mg	1.4 mg	0.82 mg	1.4 mg
Vitamin B-2	1.2 mg	1.6 mg	1.26 mg	2.26 mg
Vitamin B-3	13 mg	18 mg	11.6 mg	18.4 mg
Vitamin B-6	2.0 mg	2.2 mg	1.02 mg	2.0 mg
Vitamin B-12	3.0 mcg	3.0 mcg	17.5 mcg	22 mcg
Vitamin C	60 mg	60 mg	82.4 mg	302.4 mg
Calcium	800 mg	800 mg	904 mg	1312 mg
Vitamin D†	200 IU	200 IU	—	—
Vitamin E	11.9 IU	14.9 IU	12.6 IU	18.0 IU
Folacin	400 mcg	400 mcg	280 mcg	609 mcg
Iodine†	150 mcg	150 mcg	—	—
Iron	18 mg	10 mg	12 mg	19.8 mg
Magnesium	300 mg	350 mg	172.2 mg	377.2 mg
Phosphorus	800 mg	800 mg	1330 mg	1705 mg
Protein	44 gm	56 gm	66 gm	81.3 gm
Zinc	15 mg	15 mg	13.1 mg	18.4 mg

Nutrient values of daily menus were calculated with Health-Aide nutrition software, Programming Technology Corporation, San Rafael, California, 1982.

* The Recommended Dietary Allowances (RDA) are taken from Committee on Dietary Allowances, Food and Nutrition Board, *Recommended Dietary Allowances* (ninth revised edition), Washington, D.C. Complete information for age groups other than those listed here, and for pregnant or lactating women, may be found on page 291.

† Nutrient values for vitamin D and iodine are indeterminate, but it is very unlikely that anyone will get less than the full RDA daily if milk or fish is included in the diet.

gm = gram   IU = international unit   mcg = microgram   mg = milligram

The Pocket Diet: Other Important Nutritional Needs

Nutrient	Recommendation*	Daily Average Supplied by Diet		Comment†
		Basic Diet, No Additions	Total with Soup Addition	
Calories	Varies	988	1233	Add treats or needs or both to bring calories to desired level
Carbohydrates	Approximately 58% total calories	114 gm	164 gm	Carbohydrates = about 53% daily calories
Crude Fiber	6 gm or more	7 gm	13.5 gm	Strain the soup if it has too much roughage for you
Potassium	1875–5625 mg	2539 mg	4860 mg	Stay on the high side
All Fats‡	Not to exceed 30% total calories	32 gm	34.1 gm	
Saturated	Approximately 10% total calories	9 gm	9.1 gm	Fats = 25% daily calories (7% saturated, 7.5% monounsaturated, 2% polyunsaturated)
Monounsaturated	Approximately 10% total calories	10 gm	10.3 gm	
Polyunsaturated	Approximately 10% total calories	3 gm	3 gm	
Cholesterol	300 mg maximum	184 mg	194 mg	Keep on the low side
Sodium	1100–3300 mg maximum	982 mg	1268 mg	Keep on the low side
Sugar	Not to exceed 10% total calories	0.8 gm	0.8 gm	Sugar = less than 1% daily calories

Nutrient values of daily menus were calculated with Health-Aide nutrition software, Programming Technology Corporation, San Rafael, California, 1982.

* Nutrient Recommendations regarding carbohydrates, fats, cholesterol, and sugar are part of the Dietary Goals for the United States, prepared by the Senate Select Committee on Nutrition and Human Needs, 1977. Other recommendations are broad guidelines as reported in *Recommended Dietary Allowances.*

† Percentages are based on total with soup addition.

‡ Because values are not available for some minor fatty acids, the amounts listed in each group do not add up to the total for all fats.

Customizing the Diet

CALCULATING CALORIE NEEDS

1. Enter here your daily calorie needs or goals: _____
   (Use the table on page 50, or follow the guidelines in
   Chapter 12 for finding your personal balance. Remember, for best health results, women should generally consume no fewer than 1200 calories daily, and
   men no fewer than 1500, for any extended period.)
2. This is the average daily number of calories in the
   basic diet, without additions: 988
3. Subtract step 2 from step 1 to learn how many additional calories daily you will require, on average: _____

FILLING YOUR NEEDS: SOME SUGGESTIONS

1. As shown in the nutrient analysis tables, adding *half* the High-
   Nutrient Soup recipe (see page 228) *daily* completes virtually
   all nutritional requirements while adding just 245 calories per
   day. (You'll probably want to use the soup vegetables as finger
   foods.) If you choose not to use the High-Nutrient Soup, the
   lists in Food Sources of Major Nutrients, Chapter 17, will help
   you select foods to meet your nutritional needs. You could, for
   example, forgo the soup and instead add these foods daily:

   ¼ cup wheat germ
   ¼ cup wheat bran
   1 cup raw mushrooms
   1 cup cooked beets
   1 cup raw zucchini
   2 small bananas

   Women will need to add another daily source of iron, such
   as 1 cup parsley or 2 cucumbers, to meet the RDA.
   To meet vitamin B-1 requirements, men should also add 2
   tablespoons wheat germ or other B-1 food.
2. Even with the soup, men will need to add a B-6 food; 1 small
   banana every other day would meet the RDA.
3. Once your nutrient needs are taken care of, you can add other
   foods you like to bring your calorie intake to the desired level.
   The lists in Chapter 14 will help you make good choices.

IF YOU MUST EAT FROM CANS AND BOTTLES

Fresh is best, but when you can't avoid using prepared foods, remember these tips.

Do not store unfinished portions in cans. Transfer to glass containers and store in refrigerator whenever possible.

> Underwood liver paste
> Grossingers chopped liver (fat added; use sparingly)
> tomato paste — unsalted
> V-8 juice — unsalted
> peanut butter — nothing added
> fruit packed in white grape juice
> fruit juice — nothing added

If you can find them, buy these only unsalted. So far my search has been unsuccessful. Do not rinse! You lose nutrients. Save any fluids you drain off for use in soups.

soy beans	lima beans	chickpeas
kidney beans	black beans	navy beans

I'm hoping the day will come when all these foods will be canned in water, without salt.

mackerel	shrimp	lobster
sardines	oysters	crab
salmon		

I still want to see all these foods in vacuum-packed dark glass jars with threaded lids, or else in cans that state "nonaluminum surfaces" and "cans not sealed with lead."

I still want a way to prevent threads of aluminum landing in the food, and further, improved can openers that would not get clogged with bacteria-ridden residues of food that are hard to clean away. Maybe we should have throwaway, one-time-use can openers or key-type openers like those on some sardine cans. The manufacturers have done it for soft drinks, why not food? And of course we want "Nutritional Ingredients" and "Non-Nutritional Ingredients" labeling on all products sold as food.

How Is the Diet Going?

The checklists and chart will help you keep track of how you're feeling and how you're doing on this diet. Paying close attention to your body's signals may help you determine whether this is the diet for you.

The Pocket Diet:
Daily Checklist of Negative and Positive Factors

	DAY									
NEGATIVE FACTORS	1	2	3	4	5	6	7	8	9	10
Constipated										
Diarrhea										
Sleepless										
Irritable										
Itchy										
Sneezing										
Hungry										
Headache										
Blackout										
Gas										
Heartburn										
Bloat										
Weakness										
Fatigue										
Nervous										
Anxious										
Tremors										

POSITIVE FACTORS

Bowel movement *										
Sleeping well										
Stomach satisfied										
Alert, clear-headed										
Feel strong										
Lively										

* 1–3 times/day with regular, well-formed stool

The Pocket Diet: Daily Weight Change Chart

The horizontal line through the middle of the chart represents your starting weight (Day 1). Each day, mark a new point to show how your weight is changing (or not) as the diet progresses. Draw a line from point to point to chart your weight change.

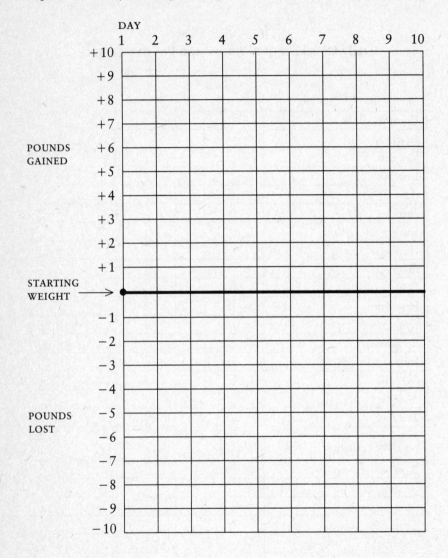

❧ 11 ❧

The Lean,
Clean Machine Diet

The Lean, Clean Machine Diet is to help flush the body of excesses. It contains practically no fats, no cholesterol, few calories or carbohydrates, and little sodium.

On the other hand, this diet contains lots of water, potassium, calcium, magnesium, virtually all necessary nutrients, and more than enough fiber (but you can strain it out if you need to) to keep you healthy. If you are sick and tired of fighting weight gains and losses over which you seem to have little control, this diet almost guarantees you success with a minimum of effort.

There are no choices to make. Just the same good soup for anywhere from a few days to as long as you want. Use good judgment. This diet is not meant for those already the right weight unless it is just for a day or two to settle an unsettled system. It is not meant to be used alone over extended periods of time. No sensible person would use this diet as an excuse to indulge in excesses throughout the week, though if you are forced into lunch and dinner meetings constantly, this soup may be a way to keep yourself healthy in spite of those usually disastrous meals.

You will not suffer from hunger pangs on the High-Nutrient Soup. The fiber- and nutrient-rich broth is quite filling. It really is surprising just how satisfying this diet is.

Full Nutrition from One Pot of Soup

For the Lean, Clean Machine Diet to provide a full complement of nutrients, there are three foods that must be added to the basic vegetable broth in rotation eight of the ten days of the diet: wheat germ, liver (any kind, bought only from health food store—clean sources), and oysters (fresh or canned, but not smoked). These three foods help you to meet the requirements for zinc, vitamin B-12, and vitamin E. The foods can be put through the blender with a small amount of the broth and then added back to the pot of soup.

Those of you who may have a serious dislike for any of these foods might like to know that in these amounts you are not going to taste them in the soup. I am sure that some of you will prefer to go to supplements to fill these nutrient discrepancies. Recognize that this is your choice, not a necessity. If you have any kind of an underlying condition for which your doctor has designed your diet, stay with that diet until receiving his or her approval to make a change.

This diet is made up of nutritionally rich foods that naturally contain few calories. In fact, almost everyone will need to *add* other foods to the diet in order to meet their calorie needs. At fewer than 500 calories daily, the soup recipe should *not* constitute your sole food intake except under close medical supervision. Nonetheless, by meeting virtually all your nutritional needs in a very small number of calories, the Lean, Clean Machine Diet is the perfect base for any weight-loss plan as well as an outstanding *natural* nutritional supplement. (This is why we recommend that the High-Nutrient Soup accompany the other diets in this book.) No worries about eating too much of the Lean, Clean Machine Diet!

Some Suggestions If You Choose This Diet

If you have digestive problems that preclude your using the rough-age, which is high in this diet because of the soup vegetables, you can use just the strained broth. Be sure to press *all* the liquid from the vegetables so you won't miss any nutrients.

If you have problems with chewing because of tooth or gum problems, you could use strained broth, but consider instead putting the soup through the blender to puree it in small batches. This preserves the roughage, which for most of us is very important to keep or even to increase in our diet.

Some people have a tendency to have food show up in rather large shreds in their stool. This is obviously a sign that their digestion is not as good as it might be or that they bolt their food. Chewing thoroughly helps, but if you can't chew well, pureeing is a good way to maximize food surfaces, making them open to digestion.

Purists or those who are using the Raw Diet besides the Lean, Clean Machine Diet might want to put the raw vegetables through a juicer and use the straight juice, or they might want to mix the raw vegetable juices with distilled water for a slightly extended soup. If you want the juices cold, put the vegetables in the refrigerator before you juice them. There is no doubt at all that vegetable juices are better immediately after juicing. Do small batches often, if you can. If you don't own a juicer, you can put small amounts of the vegetables at a time through the blender with a little distilled or spring water and even add a few herbs (fresh herbs are wonderful) to make it even better. This variation makes delicious quick soups good enough for guests. You choose whether to serve them raw or cooked.

The Lean, Clean Machine Diet is both the full nutritional base for all the other diets and a wonderful "cleaning up" diet for your body for weekends and vacations.

Shopping List

The items listed are those needed to prepare the nutrient-rich soup plus the recommended additions. All these foods are necessary to complete the daily menus.

VEGETABLES	OTHER	
celery	liver, any kind (package	oysters (package
green beans	in ⅛-pound pieces to	separately to freeze)
parsley	freeze)	wheat germ (keep
scallions		refrigerated)
zucchini		

Daily Menus

The High-Nutrient Soup

The High-Nutrient Soup, which makes up this diet, centers on the Basic High-Potassium Soup described in detail on page 228. The recipe given there provides the base for one day's quantity of High-Nutrient Soup; you may choose to use a greater or lesser volume of liquid in preparing the soup, but the vegetable ingredients should be used in the quantities listed.

These are the additions that *must* be made to the Basic Soup each day if the Lean, Clean Machine Diet is to fulfill the RDA for the ten-day period:

Day 1 — Add one oyster.
Day 2 — Add ¼ cup wheat germ.
Day 3 — Add ⅛ pound liver.
Day 4 — Add one oyster.
Day 5 — Add ¼ cup wheat germ.
Day 6 — Soup without additions.
Day 7 — Add one oyster.
Day 8 — Add ¼ cup wheat germ.
Day 9 — Add ⅛ pound liver.
Day 10 — Soup without additions.

Nutrient Analysis

These tables show the average daily nutrients supplied by the Lean, Clean Machine Diet so you can see how they compare with standard recommendations. Figures include the nutrients provided by the basic diet as listed in the daily menus, and the nutrients supplied if an extra half-portion of the High-Nutrient Soup is used as a supplement. The averages are based on the ten-day total for each nutrient, and the figures have been rounded off. (For a fuller discussion of what the figures mean, turn to page 49.)

The Lean, Clean Machine Diet: Meeting Your Needs for Nutrients Having Established RDA *

| | RDA | | Daily Average Supplied by Diet | |
| | Woman Aged 23–50 | Man Aged 23–50 | Basic Diet, No Additions | Total with Extra Soup |
Nutrient				
Vitamin A	4000 IU	5000 IU	20,080 IU	30,120 IU
Vitamin B-1	1.0 mg	1.4 mg	1.1 mg	1.7 mg
Vitamin B-2	1.2 mg	1.6 mg	2.0 mg	3.0 mg
Vitamin B-3	13 mg	18 mg	13.6 mg	20.4 mg
Vitamin B-6	2.0 mg	2.2 mg	2.0 mg	3.0 mg
Vitamin B-12	3.0 mcg	3.0 mcg	9.1 mcg	13.6 mcg
Vitamin C	60 mg	60 mg	439 mg	659 mg
Calcium	800 mg	800 mg	816 mg	1224 mg
Vitamin D†	200 IU	200 IU	—	—
Vitamin E	11.9 IU	14.9 IU	10.9 IU	16.3 IU
Folacin	400 mcg	400 mcg	659 mcg	988 mcg
Iodine†	150 mcg	150 mcg	—	—
Iron	18 mg	10 mg	15.6 mg	23.4 mg
Magnesium	300 mg	350 mg	410 mg	615 mg
Phosphorus	800 mg	800 mg	750 mg	1125 mg
Protein	44 gm	56 gm	30.6 gm	45.9 gm
Zinc	15 mg	15 mg	10.6 mg	15.9 mg

Nutrient values of daily menus were calculated with Health-Aide nutrition software, Programming Technology Corporation, San Rafael, California, 1982.

* The Recommended Dietary Allowances (RDA) are taken from Committee on Dietary Allowances, Food and Nutrition Board, *Recommended Dietary Allowances* (ninth revised edition), Washington, D.C. Complete information for age groups other than those listed here may be found on page 291. This diet is not recommended for pregnant or lactating women.

† Nutrient values for vitamin D and iodine are indeterminate, but it is very unlikely that anyone will get less than the full RDA daily if milk or fish is included in the diet.

gm = gram   IU = international unit   mcg = microgram   mg = milligram

The Lean, Clean Machine Diet: Other Important Nutritional Needs

Nutrient	Recommendation*	Daily Average Supplied by Diet		Comment†
		Basic Diet, No Additions	Total with Extra Soup	
Calories	Varies	491	736	Add treats or needs or both to bring calories to desired level
Carbohydrates	Approximately 58% total calories	100 gm	150 gm	Carbohydrates = about 81% daily calories; you may want to add protein foods
Crude Fiber	6 gm or more	13 gm	19.5 gm	If this is too much roughage, strain the soup or consume some vegetables as juice
Potassium	1875–5625 mg	4642 mg	6963 mg	Stay on the high side
All Fats‡	Not to exceed 30% total calories	4.3 gm	6.4 gm	Fats = 8% daily calories (less than 1% saturated, 1% monounsaturated, 0% polyunsaturated); this very low level allows you to add such foods as meats, fish, nuts in moderation without exceeding limits
Saturated	Approximately 10% total calories	0.14 gm	0.2 gm	
Monounsaturated	Approximately 10% total calories	0.63 gm	0.9 gm	
Polyunsaturated	Approximately 10% total calories	0 gm	0 gm	
Cholesterol	300 mg maximum	20 mg	30 mg	Will increase if high-protein foods are added
Sodium	1100–3300 mg maximum	572 mg	858 mg	Keep on the low side
Sugar	Not to exceed 10% total calories	0 gm	0 gm	

Nutrient values of daily menus were calculated with Health-Aide nutrition software, Programming Technology Corporation, San Rafael, California, 1982.

* Nutrient Recommendations regarding carbohydrates, fats, cholesterol, and sugar are part of the Dietary Goals for the United States, prepared by the Senate Select Committee on Nutrition and Human Needs, 1977. Other recommendations are broad guidelines as reported in *Recommended Dietary Allowances.*

† Percentages are based on total with extra soup.

‡ Because values are not available for some minor fatty acids, the amounts listed in each group do not add up to the total for all fats.

Customizing the Diet

CALCULATING CALORIE NEEDS
1. Enter here your daily calorie needs or goals: _____
    (Use the table on page 50, or follow the guidelines in
    Chapter 12 for finding your personal balance. Remember, for best health results, women should generally
    consume no fewer than 1200 calories daily, and men
    no fewer than 1500, for any extended period of time.
    This diet is not recommended for pregnant or lactating
    women because of its economy of calories.)
2. This is the average daily number of calories in the
    basic diet, without additions: 491
3. Subtract step 2 from step 1 to learn how many additional calories daily you will require, on average: _____

FILLING YOUR NEEDS: SOME SUGGESTIONS
1. As shown in the nutrient analysis tables, increasing the High-
    Nutrient Soup recipe by 50 percent *daily* completes nearly all
    nutritional requirements while adding just 245 calories per
    day. If you choose not to increase the soup recipe, the lists in
    Food Sources of Major Nutrients, Chapter 17, will help you
    select foods to meet your nutritional needs. You could, for
    example, forgo the extra soup and round out nutrient requirements by adding these foods to the daily diet:

    > ½ tablespoon safflower or sesame oil
    > 1 cup raw mushrooms
    > 4 ounces chicken, turkey, or fish (men use 6 ounces)
    > 1 oyster or other zinc source

    Women who choose not to use the oyster should be sure to
    add some iron-rich equivalent daily to meet the RDA. Men
    should add a B-1 source (such as 1 cup peas) daily, and a B-6
    source (1 cup tomato juice or 1 banana, for example).
2. Even if the soup quantity is increased, men will need to add
    protein to the diet. One-quarter pound turkey breast or its
    equivalent daily would meet the RDA.
3. Once your nutrient needs are taken care of, you can add other
    foods you like to bring your calorie intake to the desired level.
    The lists in Chapter 14 will help you make good choices.

How Is the Diet Going?

The checklists and chart will help you keep track of how you're feeling and how you're doing on this diet. Paying close attention to your body's signals may help you determine whether this is the diet for you.

The Lean, Clean Machine Diet: Daily Checklist of Negative and Positive Factors

NEGATIVE FACTORS	DAY 1	2	3	4	5	6	7	8	9	10
Constipated										
Diarrhea										
Sleepless										
Irritable										
Itchy										
Sneezing										
Hungry										
Headache										
Blackout										
Gas										
Heartburn										
Bloat										
Weakness										
Fatigue										
Nervous										
Anxious										
Tremors										

POSITIVE FACTORS										
Bowel movement*										
Sleeping well										
Stomach satisfied										
Alert, clear-headed										
Feel strong										
Lively										

* 1–3 times/day with regular, well-formed stool

The Lean, Clean Machine Diet: Daily Weight Change Chart

The horizontal line through the middle of the chart represents your starting weight (Day 1). Each day, mark a new point to show how your weight is changing (or not) as the diet progresses. Draw a line from point to point to chart your weight change.

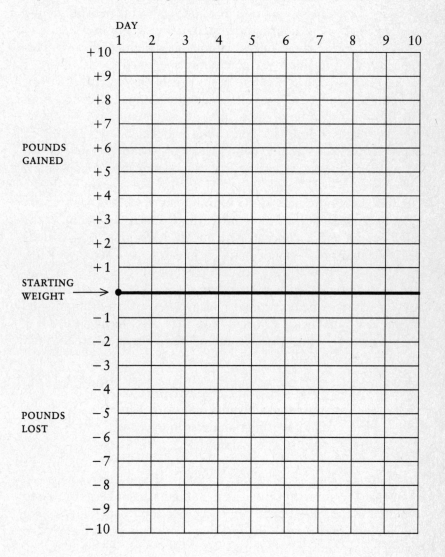

Summing Up

Raw vegetables may upset a particular individual's system, while the same vegetables put through a juicer and taken without the roughage may be drunk and digested easily. Many of the elderly find they cannot chew foods without great effort, that it takes them too long to finish the commonly suggested foods. There is no harm in mixing foods into raw or cooked vegetable or fruit juice, in a blender, to provide a nutritious liquefied concoction. The food can then be presented hot, as soup, cold, as a drink, or even frozen, as a popsicle. This can provide adequate nutrition to many people who cannot chew because of weakness, thick saliva, dentures, or disease, or for those of us who may need a single meal in a hurry.

The soup/broth/juices in the Lean, Clean Machine Diet are very light because they lack fats and carbohydrates. They are at the same time a more concentrated, highly nutritious food than is usually eaten on a regular basis by most of us. There are a few individuals who will have adverse reactions even to these foods, but because they can be prepared in a variety of ways, the problems can usually be overcome. This diet is very satisfying in spite of the low number of calories. You may miss feeling *full* for a couple of days while you accommodate to this new feeling, but you will feel satisfied.

 Every step in the digestive process should be activated on a daily basis and kept functioning as much of our life as is possible.

However, don't plan to *live* on soup. If you can chew, keep chewing. The strength of our teeth and gums is basic to our good health; the full importance of mixing our food with saliva is not well enough understood; the fact that some elements are absorbed through the mucous membranes of the mouth is not common knowledge. Every step has a function. Every step in the function of digestion is important.

The Lean, Clean Machine Diet is meant to "fill in" as well as to give a full nutritional base on a good diet. It has also been designed to provide good alternative ways to get the best nutrition for those whose systems cannot function at top level, whether it is for the moment or forever.

No diet "cures" you of anything. A good diet makes you healthier and by raising your nutritional state improves the quality of your life. And that means a lot. Allowing your nutrients to lapse magnifies any misery. The good effects that you will achieve through nutrition will not happen overnight. It takes a long time to weaken your body. It is going to take at least a few weeks to begin to see very big differences.

❧ PART III ❧

Balancing Food and Movement with the Cards

❧ 12 ❧

Eat — and Keep Moving

Say you have created an eating strategy that you like and one that also seems to like you. You have no discomfort of any kind, you feel better than you've felt in ages, you look terrific, and the diet is doing for you what you wanted done — weight control, health control, ease of use, great foods. The diets are designed so that you should be able to find a general type or group of foods that will suit best your hereditary and environmental needs.

What's next?

Continue to keep daily records while you remain on the diet for a month, two months! Note any problems, no matter how slight. In this time, most people will find that other little adjustments are needed. This can range from wanting more variety in the foods in your new diet to finding minor physical problems that you can see more clearly as your general health improves. Be aware that things other than diet might be the reason for the change.

Now it's time to see if your diet can be improved even further and fine-tuned to be much more specific in addressing your unique needs. Aided by some of the suggestions in this book, along with your own careful records, say to yourself, "The diet is working well, but I think I may need to add more of this particular kind of food or this particular nutrient." You will gain the clearest information about your progress if you make just one change at a time in your diet and continue that change for a few weeks to see if you are getting the effect you hoped you would. Remember, the human body changes slowly. You will see and feel the effects long before anyone else will notice them. Give yourself time to see the change that you are looking for take place.

You Are in Control

Your body works a little differently from anyone else's according to heredity, environment, present condition of health, daily habits, and your own idiosyncratic workings. *You* know your body best. According to how you balance your moving and your eating — and in spite of a metabolism that may seem, in the beginning, to work against you — you can gain weight, you can lose weight, you can maintain weight. You are the only one who with enough personal education can adjust your daily intake of food, your daily output of energy, till the balance is just right to maintain steady change in the direction you want.

The best way to lose weight is to balance food against activity knowledgeably. You can lose weight by doing any one of these:

- Eat less.
- Change to a better kind of food.
- Eat several smaller meals instead of one or two large meals.
- Move (or exercise) longer.
- Move (or exercise) with weights.
- Choose a more difficult form of exercise, sport, or dancing.

And you can lose weight faster by combining two, three, four, or all of the above. These are all things that are within your power to do. This is especially important when weight control is difficult to attain. Don't give up! The more problems you have with it, the greater the eventual accomplishment. Great self-confidence comes with taking control.

You have a lot to gain healthwise if you achieve a needed weight loss. And you can lose weight

- without feeling weak
- without going hungry
- without getting bad breath
- without becoming constipated

- without feeling nervous
- without getting slack or flabby
- without feeling sick
- without eating less

Do not hesitate to make choices in adapting the diets in this book to your needs. Your likes and dislikes are important if you are to stay on a diet. How you are feeling is important if you are to stay on a diet. The controls are in your hands! You must, to design your perfect diet, cut out anything you hate, anything that makes you feel ill in any way. But for the sake of your health, *never cut out the nutritional necessities.*

Keeping Track

The method I want to show you for keeping track so that you know exactly what needs changing and when, is the same system that is used for collecting systematic information on any problem. It is the daily log of what you do and what happens to you. This is the same principle used to captain a ship or run a laboratory. Our memories are not so good that we remember hourly, or daily, details that will enable us to gauge our progress over time. If we're depressed we remember mostly bad things. If we're elated we remember mostly good things. But whatever is remembered is colored by the moment. Only a faithful record written at the time shows the actual course of change. So I suggest you keep a daily record on cards so you can see how the changes you make in diet and activity seem to be related to changes you see in your health and quality of life.

Begin *right now,* even before you embark on any of the diets in this book. Believe me, the information gained will be eye-opening and will enhance your awareness of what your present habits really are. Very often a change in how you feel lags days or even weeks behind a change in habit. Especially when used along with the daily checklists and weight charts provided at the end of the diet programs, the daily cards will tell you where you are as impersonally as a mirror.

Put up with the momentary nuisance of learning to make out the cards for the sake of a whole new, better way of living. If you don't write down your entire energy intake (your food) and your entire energy output (your movements), it is too easy to forget an item — especially if you'd rather forget. In any case, we all forget when we get busy with other things. If you really want to lose that weight (or, for some of you, gain that weight), you won't forget to write down every single calorie that you take in and every single calorie that you burn off. Your health and your life are not to be taken so lightly that you can afford to consider it too much trouble to keep the cards for a month or even two.

Keeping the cards does pay off! With daily cards you see what is actually happening. None of us remembers exactly what we have eaten, what we have had to drink, after a whole day has elapsed. Write it down as you take it in! The cards, along with the other information in this book, will make you aware of

- how many calories you eat
- how much fat and oil you consume
- how many refined foods are in your diet
- how many fatty and refined foods you can dump from your diet
- whether you're getting all essential nutrients
- how you can cut unneeded calories while increasing needed nutrients
- how many calories you burn daily, on the average
- how you might arrange other comfortable or even exciting ways to burn more calories

Getting Started with the Cards

First, buy a hundred 4-by-6-inch cards or a small ring binder notebook of about the same size to help you keep a record.

Start on a fresh card each day. Write in the left column what you eat, as you eat it, and the number of calories it contains (see sample card). You will need to buy a good calorie counter from a local bookstore. You might consider something like *Nutrients in Foods* or the *Nutrition Almanac* (see Bibliography), which include information about nutrients as well as calories.

Write in the right-hand column what your activities are and the amount of time you spend at them as you go through the day. Include everything you do: sleeping, eating, sitting. Make sure you include the activities for the full twenty-four hours. Then use the chart Calories Burned in Activities on pages 198–199 to estimate how many calories you have burned. If you don't find a specific activity on the lists, look for something that seems to be similar. An educated guess is better than no entry at all.

Sample Card

Day __(1)__ Wt. today __(130)__		Date _(7/15)_ Wt. yesterday __(130)__	
Calories In		*Calories Out*	
Breakfast		8 hr. sleeping	624
black coffee	0	4 hr. sitting quietly	288
1 banana	70	4 hr. sitting writing	408
2 eggs	120	1 hr. standing quietly	90
1 danish	200	½ hr. driving	50
1 glass whole milk	160	1 hr. slow walk	288
		1 hr. cooking	162
Lunch		2½ hr. eating	210
3 oz. hamburger	186	2 hr. talking	204
½ TBSP mayonnaise	50		
lettuce, tomato	10		
1 oz. cheese	100		
white hamburger roll	150		
chips	140		
milkshake	350		
Snack			
black coffee	0		
2 doughnuts	250		
Dinner			
½ lb. broiled chicken	300		
5 spears asparagus	26		
10 french fries	137		
chocolate cake	360		
Total Calories In:	2609	Total Calories Out:	2324

The cards are an important part of the learning process. Some people have to look at and work with the cards longer than others before they finally begin to change their habits in the way that is right for their body. Try to keep the cards very carefully for at least three months. You'll be surprised at how much you can learn from them. After the initial period, everyone still needs a once or twice yearly check to make sure good new habits are being maintained.

The sample card is meant to be a *bad example,* in which you would probably be gaining weight slowly but surely. This card also has many *poor food choices,* which would leave you less than well nourished.

Every individual is unique. Many "normal" differences can cause us to gain and lose weight at a rate just a little different from the rates of others — metabolic rates, muscle mass, the body's ability to handle certain foods better than others, many variables of this kind, plus differing calorie or even weight counts of foods (no two carrots weigh the same, have exactly the same number of calories or the same amount of vitamin A). Numbers given in any nutritional guide are close approximations only. Nutrition can never be an exact science. You will get a feel for your own diet, but you can never be specific.

The cards you keep may look quite improperly out of balance and yet you may be moving toward your goal, whether it's losing, maintaining, or gaining weight. It is your internal balance you are looking for. When your body reacts as you want through use of the cards, continue to use the cards till your habits are set to help you maintain the improvements.

Seeking the Proper Balance

On the right-hand side of your 4-by-6 card or notebook, write down all the moving, sitting, and sleeping that you do, starting with your hours of sleep first thing in the morning and continuing with all your activities throughout the day.

On the left-hand side write down everything that passes your lips: meals, drinks, gum, alcoholic beverages, tastes, snacks, breath fresheners — everything!

At the end of each day total up each of the two columns. You will see clearly the trash you eat, the calories consumed, how much you sit. Take heart! It helps you to start changing immediately.

Now you must begin to listen closely to what the cards are telling you. If you are trying to lose weight, you will probably have to learn to arrange your life so that the food intake calories are always lower than the energy output calories. (For some people the balance is quite different.) If you keep the activities column at just the right level for *you*, you're going to be losing weight. You will be able to tell, once you've adjusted to the point that you are losing weight (or gaining weight, if that is your goal), where your balance comes. Just like a tightrope walker, you'll find that with time and practice balancing becomes easy. Hard to believe now, maybe, but true nonetheless. In fact, once you have lost the weight you want, you will have to adjust the balance again to keep from losing too much. And for those who are working at gaining weight, the balancing act is just as important. (You'll find more about analyzing your cards in Chapter 13.)

According to body weight, energy level, metabolism, length of limbs, amount of muscle tissue, and a number of other criteria, every person who performs a particular activity will use up a different number of calories than another person performing that same activity. The calories used may be only roughly in the same ballpark.

Because you are unique in your use of calories, if you are trying to lose weight you may find a balance that looks as if you must try to work or play very hard. You may not have the time, energy, or inclination for this kind of lifestyle. You can choose instead to change your food intake. Just be sure the necessities — all the nutrients — are covered.

Does Physical Activity Really Burn Calories? Yes, and More!

When we get too much of any food, except some vegetables, we convert it and lay it away as fat. Fat is stored energy, very much like gas in the tank of a car. At any given moment a little bit of gas is being converted into the power that runs the car; the rest is in the tank. Your body converts stored fat into the power to run your body *only* when there are not enough needed sugars immediately available. If you are taking in foods that provide those sugars at regular intervals, the stored fat either just sits there or continues to grow from excess foodstuffs that you eat. You become a fuel storage tank on legs. If you try to put too much gas in the tank of a car it will overflow. Our big problem is that our bodies do not overflow. We just keep filling all our little tanks, called fat cells, till we can barely move.

One pound of fat is between 3500 and 4000 calories. To rid yourself of one pound of stored fat, you have three alternatives:

1. You must be active enough so that over a period of days your particular metabolism will burn more than 3500 calories over and above what you normally use daily in your activities at this time. For each person, losing weight is just a little different. It may be a little harder for you to work off that number of calories. If you choose your form of activity wisely and increase gradually the amount of time and effort spent at it, working it off can give you a slow, safe, and steady loss of weight and some terrific benefits. But exercise by itself is not really to be preferred, since you will not get all the same benefits you would get from a combination of excellent diet and exercise.

2. You can achieve the same weight goal by lowering your daily intake of calories so that over a period of days you consume about 3500 fewer calories than usual. If at the same time you also increase your nutrient intake, this can be wonderful for improving your nutritional health. But it is not really to be preferred by itself, since you will miss the benefits you would get from exercise.

3. For the greatest success story you should both increase the number of calories burned and decrease the number of calories consumed while improving the nutrient value in your diet. This is a terrific alternative! You are giving yourself the opportunity to lose weight twice as fast, to gain health twice as fast, and to look twice as good!

The diet strategies in this book insure that your health will be improved by the better foods and the lessening of caloric intake. And with the use of the information on calorie burning and exercise found in the charts later in this chapter, you can devise an exercise strategy that will assure you of increased and improved circulation and an ever more efficient metabolism, which will help you to burn more calories. As you increase the amount of time spent at easy activities or develop over a period of time ever more strenuous activities, your metabolism will improve even more. Obviously, before embarking on any very different exercise program, it is sensible to discuss it with your physician. Be smart. Prevent possible problems, which will slow your progress.

Exercise means more to you than just a few extra calories burned. For instance, you cannot diet away the looseness of muscles. You must exercise to tighten the muscles, to make them look lean and streamlined. Many people will tell you that there is no such thing as "spot" exercises, yet women by the dozens have lost inches from their hips in the classes in Self-Designed Fitness that I directed at the Massachusetts Institute of Technology, not from

---

YOU MAY GAIN ALL THIS AND MORE
FROM PHYSICAL ACTIVITY

Your body firms up.
Circulation improves.
Endurance improves.
Skin color improves.
Your skin tone improves.
Aches and pains tend to diminish.
You feel less tired.
You lose weight faster.
Your blood pressure tends to normalize.
You sleep better.
Your breathing improves.
Your joints move more smoothly.
Muscles smooth and tighten.
You can lose inches where you want.
You can gain inches where you want.
You work off tensions.
You feel much more cheerful.
You feel much more confident.
Your body's entire assortment of systems feels more
    synchronized.

losing weight but by the daily repetition of one single, very efficient exercise to tighten up extremely slack muscles. One woman, who will always stand out in my mind, lost from her hips (which she thought were hereditarily enormous) a full seven inches over a year's time. She did *not* lose weight! In fact, I have dealt with many anorexics who are trying to get rid of slack bellies and thighs with weight loss when their problem comes from nutrition so poor that the body cannot maintain the muscles in a slick, tight condition.

With physical activity you can do away with excess water weight, fat, and slack muscles (called flab). But you can diet away only the water and the fat. The right diet can make you feel more energetic and can elicit better contractions from the muscles. But only physical activity will really develop the muscles to their full capacity.

Make Double Use of Time

People who are extremely sedentary often think physical activity must of necessity take more time out of their lives. But increasing your level of activity doesn't have to take more time, if that is what is in short supply for you.

Nowadays you constantly see people walking or running with friends and colleagues, visiting as they move; or working out with business associates at the local health spa (as they've always played golf), discussing as they get a little or a lot of exercise; or walking or running stairs in their office buildings instead of waiting for elevators, developing muscles and improving circulation even as they save waiting time.

More important is what I have watched played out many times to my satisfaction. Within a few weeks of beginning to exercise, whether in exercise classes, weightlifting, sports, dancing — whatever gets a person moving — almost everyone comments on sleeping better and many speak of needing fewer hours of sleep. In our classes, many have found their requirement for sleep cut as much as in half. And invariably after a period of leaping around stirring your circulation, taking a break from possibly more sedentary occupations, you will go back to your regular work refreshed in both mind and body. You will work better after exercise in almost every case.

What Kind of Physical Activity? How?

Choose the form of exercise that you need or that you feel you will continue. If what you choose is done consistently you will not only lose weight much more efficiently but also lose that weight more effectively. You will be choosing not just to lose weight but to have your body look a lot better than it can by diet alone, and you will be choosing to get your body to work a lot better.

I have met many people who thought they needed to lose weight when all they required was improved posture and tighter muscles. I know many people who with exercise alone have lost so many inches that they have appeared twenty pounds lighter in a year's time.

Please start exercise of any sort gradually. Overenthusiasm has ruined more programs than you can imagine. And those same people will decide never to try again because they started foolishly. Ever done that? You're supposed to *learn* by your mistakes how to do things the *right* way, not stop entirely because you *didn't* choose to move wisely in the first place.

And, please, don't believe warming up and cooling down are for the rest of the world. Many injuries, much pain and stiffness result from lack of sensible, gradual starting-up and slowing-down routines.

Now all you need is desire — your motivation, your determination. Your body is very adaptable and it can, to a large extent, turn into whatever kind of body you want it to be, if you're willing to put in the effort. Maybe you have tried before. If you didn't succeed, maybe it's because you didn't try the right way! Didn't choose the right activity. Try again — and again and again if necessary.

Just don't stop trying till you've got the results that you want!

Work and Play and the Energy Equation

The charts that follow will help you calculate the calories in-calories out balance that works for you. But remember that the numbers in the charts are *average numbers only!* The values are included to help you to begin to determine your approximate daily

Activity	Body Weight				
	110 lb.	*130 lb.*	*150 lb.*	*170 lb.*	*190 lb.*
Easy Living					
lying at ease	11	13	15	17	19
cooking (F)	23	27	31	35	39
cooking (M)	24	28	33	37	41
eating	12	14	16	18	20
sitting writing	15	17	20	22	25
sitting quiet	11	12	14	16	18
standing quietly (F)	13	15	17	19	22
standing quietly (M)	14	16	18	21	23
cleaning (F)	31	37	42	48	53
cleaning (M)	29	34	39	45	50
walking, normal pace	41	48	56	63	71
Playing—Easy to Hard					
Bicycling					
leisure (5.5 mph)	32	38	44	49	55
leisure (9.4 mph)	50	59	68	77	86
racing	85	100	115	130	145
Dancing					
aerobic, medium	52	61	70	79	89
aerobic, intense	67	79	92	104	116
ballroom	26	30	35	39	44
"twist," "wiggle"	52	61	70	79	89
Circuit Training					
Hydra Fitness	66	78	90	102	114
Universal	58	69	79	89	100
Nautilus	46	55	63	71	80
free weights	43	50	58	66	74
Running					
11 min. 30 sec./mile	68	80	92	105	117
8 min./mile	108	125	142	160	177
5 min./mile	145	171	197	223	249
Swimming					
treading fast	85	100	116	131	146
treading slow	31	37	42	48	53

(Numbers for all other swimming strokes fall between these two.)

Calories Burned in Activities

◀ **Calories Expended in Ten Minutes**
Multiply each number by 6 to get calories per hour. Lying down for an hour uses 6 times 11, or 66 calories for a 110-pound person. So for an eight-hour night's sleep, the total would be 8 times 66, or 528 calories, and a third of the day is accounted for. (I find it significant that the only activity in which males use fewer calories than females is in Cleaning.)

Calories Expended in One Hour of Work
Add the calories from your type of work to your hours of easy living and your play. As you can see, it pays to choose your work and play wisely!

Activity	Body Weight				
	110 lb.	*130 lb.*	*150 lb.*	*170 lb.*	*190 lb.*
bakery (F)	108	126	147	162	180
carpentry, gen.	157	186	210	240	270
coal mining (est.)	288	342	390	444	672
drawing, standing	108	126	144	168	186
electrical work	174	204	234	270	300
farming (est.)	222	258	300	342	378
forestry (est.)	294	444	516	582	648
gardening (est.)	276	324	378	426	474
machine tool work	180	210	240	270	306
mail delivery (est.)	282	330	378	432	480
musician (est.)	120	138	162	186	210
plaster, scrape, paint	192	222	258	294	324
shoe repair	138	162	186	210	234
steel mill work	372	438	504	576	642
tailoring	138	162	186	210	234
tennis instructor	330	384	444	504	564
typing	90	102	120	138	156
window cleaner (M)	174	204	234	270	307
writing	90	102	120	132	150

Source: Adapted from McArdle, W. D., Katch, F. I., and Katch, V. S., *Exercise Physiology*, Lea & Febiger, Philadelphia, 1986. Data from Bannister, E. W., and Brown, S. R., "The Relative Energy Requirements of Physical Activity," in H. B. Falls (ed.), *Exercise Physiology*, Academic Press, New York, 1968; Howley, E. T., and Glover, M. E., "The Caloric Costs of Running and Walking One Mile for Men and Women," *Medicine and Science in Sports* 6:235, 1974; Passmore, R., and Durnin, J. V. G. A., "Human Energy Expenditure," *Physiological Reviews* 35:801, 1955. Used by permission of Lea & Febiger.

energy expenditure, but they do not include the important influence of your own basal metabolism or take into account how particular foods influence your rate of calorie burning. The numbers given allow for an average basal metabolism.

There are other factors affecting the way you burn calories, such as:

- weight (overweight, except when it's muscle, really tends to slow you down — sometimes even then)
- height (taller people have a mechanical disadvantage)
- sex (men generally are more heavily muscled and have a greater respiratory capacity)
- body composition (light, medium, or heavily muscled)
- body condition (eighteen and vital or eighty and ailing, and everything in between)
- environmental conditions (such as temperature, humidity, altitude)
- whether the activity is practiced or new (new is clumsy and uses more energy)
- intensity of activity (increasing your level of energy output on a regular basis keeps calorie burning high)
- how often you engage in activities (the rate of calorie burning stays up for some time following any activity)

Believe your body! If what you are doing for it doesn't feel right, change it! Whether the problem arises in the dieting or in the exercising, there are variations to fill the most extraordinary needs, and you will find many of those variations mentioned in this book. For instance, you don't need to do violence to your body to get excellent results. Walking a half hour a day, all by itself, can bring about a loss of ten pounds in a year. Do it longer or faster or up stairs, to lose more weight, more quickly. If you can't see, you can sit on an exercise bike or walk in place holding on to the back of a chair. I know people who do. I once got a young boy with serious balance problems started riding a three-wheeled bike. It gave him both freedom of movement and the activity he needed. If you don't have any legs, there are now bicycles that can be powered by the arms, and of course we have all been inspired by those who engage in wheelchair basketball and marathons.

Trial and Error

There is no need to make a big problem of learning how to live well. Even if you eat too much, you can choose the right kinds of foods and you can learn how to work off the excess most effectively. Working it off doesn't have to be difficult. Put a rocking chair in front of the television and over a six- or eight-hour period you can burn off a significant number of calories. That may sound horrible, but many of us are already spending that much time in just that spot. If you are one of those people, try an exercise bike or a rowing machine or any of a variety of exercise aids in front of the television. You could be beautiful in no time (or exhausted). It is that simple.

> **As long as your food input level remains too high for your energy output level, you will continue to gain weight! Make your energy output level enough higher than your food intake and you will lose weight and you will begin to look both tight and slim.**

Count your day-by-day successes, no matter how small. They all add up, the same way the excesses did. Expect a few mistakes. Trial and error is the way we all learn. You've seen lots of babies learning how to walk. And a lot of tears when they've fallen, time after time after time. Did you ever see one decide it wasn't worth the effort? Losing weight doesn't happen miraculously; you have to start thinking about what you are doing as you go along. Write down what both works for you and will be good for your health over a long period of time. Start developing a plan.

It's easy to see with your daily record cards how you can greatly increase the number of calories you use up, with just a little forethought and effort. Decide on one or a few new activities that you know you would enjoy and that might even add something more to your life. Carefully, gradually increase the number of thoroughly enjoyable activities in your life, or choose activities that will give you exactly the right kind of exercise for your particular needs, whether it be endurance, slim thighs, speed, a flat belly, or all of them. Learning some new activity, one you've never tried before, takes more effort and brings more muscles into use than if you continue activities you are already practiced in. Practice makes perfect and doesn't burn as many calories.

You have in this book an enormous number of ideas about movement and diet from which you can pick and choose. Take your time. Experiment, but do it carefully and safely. Find out all kinds of things about your body and how it works. Write it all down. Keep it safe. It can be useful to you for all the rest of your life.

❧ 13 ❧

Changing Habits for a New Balance

All of us have a mixture of good and bad habits. There is also the *lack* of good habits, like *not* beginning an exercise program or *not* flossing your teeth. Throughout this book I am trying to introduce you to the reasons for adopting different habits — new habits, better habits — that will improve the rest of your life. And I am introducing you to some clearly explained methods and suggestions to put you on the path to improved health and weight control.

Changing habits of eating and habits of movement takes time. It takes energy to change to a different type of food, to change your habits of shopping, of preparing food, to keep track, to keep a watchful eye on changes in yourself. It takes energy to choose the right type of movement for yourself in the first place, to try it out to see if it is the most comfortable and enjoyable for you (to see if you can live with it), and to change to a different type of movement if you see the need for it either now or in the future.

Give yourself time to discard bad habits and adopt good ones. *You can choose to change your habits whenever you need or want to!*

"Diet" means to prescribe or regulate the intake of food; and "regulate" means to govern constantly, in short *to make a habit of control*. "Exercise" means training or drilling for the sake of attaining proficiency; and "training or drilling" means *to make a habit of action.*

Your diet may need some changes. If you are overweight, depending on your body's ability to deal with changes, your diet may need

- to be lower in calories
- to be spread out (eaten in smaller amounts throughout the day)
- to include a different kind of food
- to be prepared differently

Your exercise program (even if it's walking, biking, or dancing) may need some changes. If you are overweight, *depending on your capabilities,* you may need

- to exercise faster
- to exercise harder
- to exercise longer
- to change to a different form of exercise that uses more muscles

Put all changes on your card! Keep track!

Your weight and health will improve much more dramatically if you choose to change all these factors. But be cautious: don't add all of them all at once. Add one change at a time. At the first sign of good results carefully add the next change.

Habits of Eating

There are many different ways of successfully changing your eating habits. You should wish for, and get, total satisfaction from your food. All the senses, and then some, should be satisfied!

All of your food should be beautifully prepared, *a feast for the eyes*.

Your food should be as spicy as you like it to be. It should both *smell and taste delicious*.

You should have differing *textures* in each meal, liquids and solids, coarse to smooth.

You should be able to keep *chewing as much as you need* to satisfy yourself.

You should be able to *keep your stomach feeling as full as you like*.

You should be able to *enjoy the sounds of a meal,* at the very least from the spooning of the soup to the crunching of the vegetables.

True satisfaction in eating comes from enough of everything — taste, texture, smells, sounds, appearance, chewing, and a full stomach! Don't lust for food, have a romance with it.

Habits of Movement

Many people love to move, but not everyone does. We all do move as long as we live, even if it's only to breathe; but not all of us consciously enjoy it. We still get up in the morning, go to the store, carry groceries home, go to work, sometimes heavy, muscular work. In some cases that is enough. Toting groceries to a fourth-floor walk-up apartment is pretty good daily exercise. Do you need *more* movement than you're getting? Maybe a *different kind* is needed to balance what you get in your daily life. If you have been badly traumatized by regular sports programs or competitive sports, try to think of movement from a different direction. What kind of movement do you positively like? Walking? Dancing? Conducting an orchestra? Practicing an instrument? Singing?

All of the forms of movement you choose *must suit you and your capabilities*. As your capabilities change, change your level of activity.

Your choice of movement should *make you feel good while being performed and better afterward,* no matter at which level you are.

Your choice of movement should be performed *where you will most enjoy it* — outside if that is the appropriate place, on a dance floor if that is better suited, or even in your own bed or bedroom.

Your choice of movement should *fill some weak spot* in your assessment of your own physical needs. Consider these:

balance	joint mobility
circulation	strength
dexterity	coordination
endurance	power
flexibility	speed
posture	breathing
agility	

And let's not forget just plain old tightening of those flabby belly, thigh, and underarm muscles.

True ease in any physical activity adds a great feeling of self-confidence besides improving the quality of your life.

Making Activity Part of Your Life

As mentioned earlier, your calorie-burning rate takes some time to slow down to a resting mode when increased by regular physical activity of any kind. This may mean that a little exercise done several times a day may cause more calories to be burned than performing your whole exercise routine at one time. This "when I can find the time" method of activity fits into many more daily schedules and is certainly the most natural and safest way to go about getting the necessary daily movement for our mostly sedentary population.

Among the growing population of people over one hundred years of age (20,000 in 1985) it appears that longevity, per se, has little to do with aerobic exercise and much more to do with regular, daily, intermittent forms of activity.

Caution!

The first marathon runner died at the end of his run. We are frequently shown on television formerly healthy individuals laid out for recovery at the end of a marathon; some of these people will need a three-month recovery period after the race. This is perhaps an extreme example, but the point is that extremes of exercise can produce severe stress. Physiologists are still exploring the short- and long-term results of joint-pounding exercises, such as running on paved roads. Cross-country running over grass and earth, though much easier on the joints, has its own hazards due to the uneven terrain.

Running improperly, or uncontrolled aerobic exercise, can be enough to wreck the joints of some. Running becomes much more dangerous for those who are overweight, which will tend to increase the impact on the feet and the strain on the circulatory system. Women in general tend to have a higher degree of joint flexibility than men, which can often mean a lack of joint control. Women who are underweight or who are putting in excessive amounts of time running can find that their menstrual periods stop and will not start again till they ease off and gain some weight.

It's important to choose an appropriate and comfortable surface for whatever activity is to be performed. Exercising of any type, even standing still, can be injurious if done directly on a concrete or marble floor, even though the floor is covered with a thick rug, and even if the injuries are not instantly visible. The marvelous shoes developed to protect us from impact as we run were needed for walking many years ago, in fact as soon as the first marble and concrete floors and concrete sidewalks came into existence. Well-built shoes that reduce impact and protect us in daily life from hard surfaces will go a long way toward keeping us on our feet and moving around comfortably over a much longer period of time. Simple walking and everyday use of our legs has seen many of us through to the century mark and beyond.

Though some regular daily activity is very important to our well-being, aerobic exercise may actually be harmful for probably 50 percent or more of our population. In many cases this can be due to a variety of joint problems, including the joints of the back, and other disease problems that may be too far advanced to permit a return to aerobic-type exercises, such as diabetes, multiple sclerosis, and others. Even simple aging, when joint tissues have thinned, can make most forms of aerobic exercises not just foolish but downright dangerous.

Enough exercise of the right sort, walking included, increases your circulation, gives your skin a nice pink glow, and gives you a feeling of euphoria. You may be dreading that movement will be drudgery, but within a week or two, if not by the end of the first period of walking, dancing, or whatever your choice of movement is, you will begin to feel the difference. Movement contributes greatly to your feeling of well-being whether or not you are losing weight, but it has an even more significant effect on anyone engaged in a weight-loss program. You don't want to end a diet looking and feeling like a bag that has been emptied. Movement helps ensure that your metabolism changes with your weight, helping you to lose more effectively.

Important note: There is burgeoning evidence of the fact that the way to preserve our blood vessels is through diet more than through *excessive* exercise.

Judge well what kind of daily activity you are capable of engaging in on a regular basis. Time spent doing the right kind of movement will certainly improve your condition and may allow you to move on to more vigorous activity in a few weeks or months.

Resist Those Late-Night Snacks

With time on our hands many of us think of food. Everything in the house is up for grabs late into the evening.

Make your evenings profitable. Do things that make you feel good and that will make you healthier or smarter; things that *don't* include eating. Set up a regular program of activities for the evenings to keep your mind off food till your habits are what they need to be. Early evenings are a good time for exercise or dancing. No matter how tired you think you are, evening activities tend to revive you and make you feel great — and virtuous. If they wake you up too much do them earlier in the evening. They're a terrific boost to your mood right after you get home from work. If you insist on sitting in front of the television set, at least buy yourself an exercise bike, a rowing machine, a treadmill, or some hand weights and a rocking chair.

Practice your resistance to eating the wrong foods till it becomes habit. It is important that every food available in your home help you stick to your good intentions. This is the time to pull out the popsicles you made yourself from unsweetened fruit juice. You know what you like and you know what you need. Fill yourself up on raw vegetables, nourishing lowfat broths, soups, or juices. Healthful snacking needn't be boring. Try very spicy low-calorie

---

LISTEN TO EVERYONE, BUT . . .

You know what you like. You know what you dislike or even hate. You know what your needs are. You know in what ways you differ from your family and friends. There is no way that a particular diet will work for everyone.

Listen to everyone — *but do what you think is best.* To develop habits of eating and moving that you will stick with, you must

- choose from a very large list of excellent foods, those that you find terrific and satisfying and that make your body work as you want it to
- choose activities you are absolutely and totally enthusiastic about

Keep your activities at just the right level in relation to your food intake and you will gain, lose, build, or maintain as *you* choose. You are truly unique and, to a very large extent, you are truly capable of designing your own health and beauty strategy.

dressings with raw vegetables. Add exotic herbs, hot peppers, or caraway seed to your soups.

Evenings are the hardest time for many people who are trying to change their eating habits. Think about the evening ahead of time. Plan it! Don't just let it happen. Get it under your control.

What Is the Right Weight?

Even the right weight is a little different for each individual. There are many people who seem to be in exactly the right condition and present a very good appearance in clothes, but prove to be soft and flabby when out of their clothes. There are some who appear heavy and cumbersome in their clothes but are muscular and healthy-looking out of their clothes.

The "right weight" is not the important issue. For two healthy people of the same height and more or less the same bone structure (bones increase in weight and thickness as your muscles develop), weight can vary as much as twenty pounds or more. So the right weight is relative. What is terrific for one person could ruin the career or the health of another. Imagine an overweight pregnant woman or dancer or an underweight dockworker or body builder.

Your particular needs are important! The right weight for you may be on the light side, to adjust to a slight frame and an inherited lightly muscled body, or it may be heavy, to account for an inherited heavily muscled body. What you must look for, and adjust for, is the balance between the right food for you, to keep you healthy and to keep your weight as close to where you want it as you can, and some properly chosen activity, according to your condition and your desires, to keep your body as firm as possible and freely movable.

Fat or Overweight?

Many of us want to lose weight, many of us want to gain weight. There are also some of us who, though staying the right weight, see strange changes in ourselves that we really do not like or want to continue to live with. A healthy body is tight-muscled and firm-fleshed, with no extra bloat or padding (aging allows a less elastic skin to drape a bit).

First it is important to know what kind of weight you carry, and if it *is* extra weight. There is:

- fluid, or water, weight
- fat weight
- muscle weight

And then there is the weight faker—

- lack of muscle tone (loose or slack muscles that hang, giving the appearance of excess weight)

Fluid, or Water, Weight. Fluid weight is necessary to life and health but can become excessive. Excess water weight is the easiest weight to lose and is lost faster than either fat weight or muscle weight. Much water weight occurs from improper body chemistry. That improper chemistry can be hormonal, ordering the kidneys to retain water. It can be an allergic reaction or some particular sensitivity to a food or food group, such as salt and salty foods. It can be a reaction to some medication that causes you to hold excess fluids (this particular problem may or may not improve when the medication is stopped).

To lose excess water weight you can

- increase the foods that help you to get the right sodium–potassium ratio (see Chapter 15)
- decrease the salt level in your diet (see Chapter 15)
- increase your activity level, *if your condition will allow it;* this helps you to sweat off both sodium and potassium
- take hot baths or showers, if you have no problems with high blood pressure or other circulatory ailments; this will encourage temporary water loss (less safe, but widely done in northern Europe where eating highly salted fish is common, are steam baths and saunas)
- discuss with your doctor the possibility of a medication change, if a medication seems to be at the root of your problem; that is quite often a viable alternative

But you can go too far! Dehydration — too much loss of water — is more dangerous than excess water. Always keep up your fluid intake. The important point is to make sure that you are not retaining an excessive amount.

Fat Weight. Your *basic* fat weight is necessary to your life and health. It is the *excess* body fat that you want to get rid of. Excess fat comes from eating more calories than your body can use — too much food of all kinds, good, bad, and indifferent — between one meal and the next.

To lose excess fat weight you can

- increase your energy output, as we've been discussing
- decrease your energy intake by eating less and eating a better choice of foods

You will find many suggestions about the foods to add to your diet and foods to avoid later on in this chapter and in Part IV.

Muscle Weight. Muscular development is necessary to health and life but can sometimes be excessive in the eyes of the person who carries it. Muscle weight is the hardest form of excess weight to lose and the kind of excess you shouldn't *want* to lose. Gaining muscle weight is reason for congratulations for weight lifters (and their admirers and lovers), to whom any extra ounces or pounds of muscle in the right place is wonderful. A very different hormonal system encourages a greater and faster development of muscle in males than females from puberty to age forty or fifty, from which time this extra ability slowly tapers off. It is no accident that a thick, muscular body is considered attractive in men. But for those women who would choose to go along with the ideals of the fashion designers, an inherited tendency to a more than ordinarily muscular body, even when it is healthy and vibrant, can seem a burden and a constant source of embarrassment. It is wiser to change your mind than your body if this is the case. The following information is for those of you who have not yet gained that wisdom. To try to lose excess muscle weight you can

- not engage in lifting anything that weighs over ten to fifteen pounds (ten to fifteen pounds will keep muscles firm, larger muscle groups such as thighs and buttocks have to carry your body weight around and will stay firm enough with just that if you do a minimum of a mile or two a day of walking)
- avoid work or play that will cause your muscle mass to develop further

I personally would not seriously advise either of the above. Health is the most precious thing you will ever have, and *health is beauty*. Develop your own personal health with good food and good exercise. Make your particular and individual body the best it can be and be proud of its uniqueness! Change your *type* of exercise if you must. But do not deny your body as much movement as it wants and needs. Take up running sports, which tend to slim the muscles; try swimming, another sport which tends to slim everything but the shoulders; or take up dance classes or just go dancing often.

Lack of Muscle Tone. Many of us lack the self-awareness to be able to tell whether we have too much weight or too little muscle tone. An unexercised muscle softens, sags, and weakens. When measured with a tape measure your thighs, waist, and belly can all appear to be enormously large if you lack good muscle tone. They are really overly loose. The more a muscle weakens, the thinner and saggier it becomes until finally it hangs from one connection to another like a bundle of strings. It no longer supports movement as it should. It no longer takes the strain off the joints as it should. And it *looks terrible*. Worst of all for women is a sagging gluteus maximus (the sitting muscle) which, in sagging, slips to the side and looks like fat padding the upper thighs. Exercise rather than diet slims down those pads.

A well-used muscle is tight, elastic, and rounded. It tends to cling tightly to the bones to which it is connected. In fact, a well-used muscle helps to keep the bone strong by pulling at it.

Often-used muscles keep the waistline small, the thighs slender and beautifully shaped on both men and women, the underarms firm and smooth, the buttocks tight and round, and the belly flat and capable of holding your innards in. And often-used muscles can measure inches smaller than flab.

On the other hand, you can, if you choose, make some particular muscle or group of muscles larger by working with weights.

More About Muscle Tone

If you have a batch of frozen food and your freezer stops working, one method of keeping the food frozen is to wrap it in newspapers, which serve as insulation. The method works for hot substances also — to keep it hot, insulate it. Use a Thermos or put it in Styrofoam. The same holds true for your body.

It is important to your continued life and health that the core temperature of your body be maintained. Muscle tone is really tiny vibrations of the muscle that are always at play throughout your lifetime; one important reason for this is to keep your core temperature at the level required. Any contraction of muscles, no matter how small, burns fuel and liberates heat, which is measured in calories. The greater the tone, the more calories are expended. Shivering, for instance, burns many calories. When you sleep, even when you rest, your body is much quieter so core temperature tends to drop. If your body is covered by too large an insulating layer of fat these vibrations (the "tone") are less, and so the number of calories that muscle tone burns at night or when you rest decreases.

In addition, there is direct heat production (read, calorie expenditure) by the muscles and other tissues that goes on without muscle contraction. Muscles create heat; muscles burn calories.

So, the not-so-good news is: A person with more fat (insulation) will burn fewer calories, resting or sleeping.

The good news is: A person with less fat will burn more calories, resting and sleeping.

The best news is: Those who work with weights develop muscles that will burn still more calories, even resting and sleeping!

Increase Activities, Relieve Stress
Movement serves many functions. One of those functions is to relieve stress.

If you work under a lot of tension, or if you are an exceptionally nervous or excitable person, if you have responsibilities that weigh heavily on you, if you tend to worry about things whether you can change them or not, and if all this stress wipes you out, movement can be your salvation.

The right kind of movement can make you feel really comfortable so you can get back to work feeling less tense. A good hard walk, or a workout (take a friend along if you can) after your boss has bawled you out or a piece of work has fallen apart can be a very real stress release. If you're really uptight but you have a job that must be finished, just get up, lock the door, and run in place for a few minutes. During your coffee break, or at home after everyone has left, turn on the radio (use earphones and lock the door if you're at work) and dance wildly for a few crazy moments. An excellent safety valve (and ridiculously fun!). There are complex hormonal reasons for it, but it does work.

When you feel ready to "chuck it in," five minutes well spent can have your sense of humor back in working order. Even though the vigorous activity is not going to change the situation, it will still change your emotional response to the situation.

Hundreds of people attest to the fact that if you can incorporate reasonably active movement into your days on a regular basis, your entire life will take on a different perspective.

Just Walking Can Do It!
If you decide to park a mile from work (which is usually cheaper anyway) and walk the mile there and the mile back, and at lunchtime take a twenty-minute walk, and use the stairs instead of the elevators — in one year you would walk about seven hundred miles and lose about seventeen pounds! (59,500 calories!) Can you believe that as simple a thing as walking could make that big a difference to you?

I'm sure you have read something like this before, and I am equally sure you believe it. So have you incorporated a part of it into your life? You need the right shoes for both walking and climbing stairs, warmer clothes or clothes that make it easier to dress in layers, and you need to start out for work a little earlier in the morning. And while you're at it, try to take your lunchtime friends with you on your noon walk. By doing this you could lose seventeen pounds — and gain a tighter body!

You can make it easy for yourself to get into the habit.

- Buy the right clothes and shoes.
- Start by carrying your shoes, if you must, as you walk or run up and down stairs.
- Take a walk around the building to visit friends on every coffee or lunch break. Talk friends into going with you. Walk and talk every opportunity you get. *Don't sit!*

Have you ever noticed that your feet get larger as you gain weight? One of the things that often happens to people who are overweight is that their feet begin to ache. That extra weight pushes down on your feet, flattening your arches. The arch of your foot is supposed to act as a shock absorber, not a pedestal. You've got shock absorbers in your arches, shock absorbers in your knees, in the hip joints, and between every vertebra in your spine. To preserve the joint tissues that do the shock absorption, I suggest you keep your hips and knees just slightly flexed at all times. To preserve those joint tissues, walk and run so softly that you can barely hear a sound. Wear shoes with soft, thick soles and with insole material that absorbs further impact. Choose unpaved surfaces to walk or run on whenever possible.

If you have a significant amount of weight to lose, there is no need to injure yourself while you try to improve your health. If your weight is too much for your poor feet, try swimming or riding a regular or a stationary bike. The day will come when you can walk safely and comfortably again. Until then, take up activities that can be performed without stressing your feet.

Your Second Week with the Cards

At the end of your first week of keeping daily record cards, lay all the cards for the week out on the table. Check to see that you have totaled the number of calories, both for food taken in (calories in) and for activities (calories out). Now ask yourself, "Where did I go right and where did I go wrong?"

We start with the assumption that there are foods that build, repair, and maintain your body and your health. The proteins, vitamins, minerals, the roughage, fats and oils. No options here. You need all of them. But fats and oils certainly do not need to be *added* to your food, except in minute amounts for flavor; you get enough fats if you eat lean meat, poultry, fish, lowfat dairy products, even coconut and avocado. And you get enough oils if you eat fish, whole grains, or a few nuts and seeds daily. Similarly with sugar and salt, you get enough from your foods without having to add any extra.

First, go through the foods you've listed on your week's cards and find all the high-nutrient foods — the fresh fruits and vegetables, the lean meat or poultry, the fresh fish, the whole grains, the foods with no added fats or salt or sugar. Put a nice big A next to each of these foods in your lists, as has been done on the sample card.

Now that you have all the high-nutrient foods earmarked, look at the foods that are known or are suspected of giving people trouble with their weight and health. Many of them come mixed

Sample Card — A-Rated and X-Rated Foods

Day __(1)__ Wt. today __(130)__		Date _(7/15)_ Wt. yesterday __(130)__	
Calories In		*Calories Out*	
Breakfast		8 hr. sleeping	624
black coffee	0	4 hr. sitting quietly	288
A 1 banana	70	4 hr. sitting writing	408
X 2 eggs	120	1 hr. standing quietly	90
X 1 danish	200	½ hr. driving	50
X 1 glass whole milk	160	1 hr. slow walk	288
		1 hr. cooking	162
Lunch		2½ hr. eating	210
X 3 oz. hamburger	186	2 hr. talking	204
X ½ TBSP mayonnaise	50		
A lettuce, tomato	10		
X 1 oz. cheese	100		
X white hamburger roll	150		
X chips	140		
X milkshake	350		
Snack			
black coffee	0		
X 2 doughnuts	250		
Dinner			
A ½ lb. broiled chicken	300		
A 5 spears asparagus	26		
X 10 french fries	137		
X chocolate cake	360		
Total Calories In:	2609	Total Calories Out:	2324

in with, or added to the helpful foods. Wherever they are, it is important to find them. Look for all the following foods:

- *foods with refined white flour* — breads, rolls, pastries, pastas, gravies, crackers, cookies, pies, most prepared foods (canned or prepackaged), most restaurant food, etc.
- *foods with added sugar* — jams, jellies, soft drinks, cakes, pies, pastries, most prepared foods, most restaurant foods, etc.
- *foods with added salt* — most breads, pastries, crackers, lunch meats, chips, canned foods, most restaurant foods, etc.
- *foods with obvious or known fat* — choice grade meats, lunch meats, canned or fresh pâtés, most cheeses, any extra butter or margarine, most salad dressings, pastries, most sauces and gravies, most restaurant foods, etc.

As you find these foods on your cards, put a big X (in red if possible) next to each one of them.

Even when you think you're eating well, it is surprising how many foods sneak in that you really would rather not be eating. Keeping these cards makes it painfully clear — and that is the whole idea!

Let's carry it a step further. I assure you it will be startling. Total the calories you took in that were in health-building foods, those high in nutrients. (If you want to know more about these foods, you'll find many examples in the next chapter. The lists in Food Sources of Major Nutrients, Chapter 17, will also be helpful.) Next, total the calories that went into other foods: foods not naturally high in useful nutrients; foods too high in calories for the nutrients they do contain; foods that have nutrients artificially added to previously stripped whole foods; foods with too much fat, flour, salt, or sugar added to them.

Are low-nutrient, high-calorie foods the source of more than half the calories you take in? This is commonly the case, since these foods are where the fattening flours, fats, and sugars are concentrated. This makes very clear which foods you have to get rid of to bring your diet under your control.

Now that you can see clearly where a large part of the problem lies, try this! See how far you can reduce the number of red X's.

Decide which of the worst foods you eat you would not mind eating less of — or maybe even doing without completely! Think about the foods you do not want to live without; do you need them every day or every other day, or could you limit the eating of such foods to only once a week (maybe later you can make it once a month)? Think about what you're going to eat ahead of time. Write it all down at every meal as you eat. Carry the process even further. Try to replace every X food with an A food. The fewer X foods there are in your diet, the better your health will become and the easier it will be for you to maintain your weight. Generally, the more A foods there are in your diet, the better your health will be. But even good foods can be eaten to excess. (Protein, for example, is regularly eaten to excess in the United States.)

Use the A foods in soups and broths, juices and finger foods, steamed or lightly stir-fried dishes. The calories are always lower and the nutrient density always higher when these foods are prepared in ways such as those suggested in this book.

If you eat chicken, remove the skin. The younger the chicken or other animal, generally the less fat. Have only small amounts of fats at each meal. Indulge in few eggs till there is better research on cholesterol. Eat only whole-grain breads and other baked goods — get your money's worth. Sweeten your foods with fruits and fruit juices — your local health food store or supermarket is probably loaded with good products.

You must be ever watchful! Read labels even in health food stores. Lowfat, low-sugar, no-salt foods are becoming more common and are reasonably easy to find *if you look for them*. Change from whole milk to lowfat milk (or even lowfat sweet acidophilus milk to get good cultures and less fat).

You can gain the control you want over your diet. Write down the foods you eat at every meal at the time that you eat them. Total up the calories from your foods and your activities every night. Compare the early cards with the cards from later weeks to see how you're improving. Continue to keep a record for at least two or three months. It takes that long to develop any new habit.

Within limits you can change your metabolism. It will change more or less according to your age and condition. If you combine

GOOD FOODS VERSUS BAD FOODS

These changes will make it easier for you to control your health and your diet. You don't have to do it all at once! Make only the changes that are comfortable for you at this time. As you go along, you will probably want to change more. Every single step in the right direction helps.

X-Rated Foods: "Chuck 'Em"	A-Rated Foods: "Add 'Em"
canned and processed vegetables	fresh vegetables
fats, bacon, butter, lard	leanest fish, poultry, meats
oils, margarine (except as seasoning)	nuts, seeds
syrups, white sugars	fresh fruits
refined flour products	whole grains
whole milk products	nonfat and cultured milk products
most cheeses	yogurt spread, lowfat cheeses
alcohol, soft drinks	fresh fruit juices, water, herb tea
ham, salted and cured meats	fresh, lean, unmarbled meat
poultry with skin	poultry without skin
meat, well marbled	fish, all kinds
bottled sauces with salt and sugar	bottled sauces, no added salt or sugar
prepared and packaged mixes	"from scratch" foods
prepared and packaged meals	quick fresh-cooked meals

In time, you may have additions and subtractions of your own to place on these lists. You may want to get away from all bottled sauces. You may need to keep milk and grain products out of your diet due to allergies. You get to choose what is best for you.

several of the ways that have been mentioned, both in diet and in physical activity, you will reap the benefits. With a little attention of the right sort, your body gives you sure and dramatic rewards.

Your body has always been, in great part, under your control. The control should be conscious and educated.

❧ PART IV ❧

Making Your Diet Better and Better

❧ 14 ❧

"Add 'Em": The Choice Filler Foods, and More

In Chapter 13 you saw that you could improve your health and nutrition by adding A-rated foods to your diet. You may need to know more about these foods, and you may be able to use suggestions about how you can make them a habit. Included on the following pages are many of the foods and recipes referred to frequently in the daily meal plans. Whether or not you decide to build your food strategy around one or more of the eight core diets, consider seriously the daily use of these foods, especially the Choice Filler Foods: they are inexpensive, easy to prepare, low in calories, and unusually high in nutrients.

The Choice Filler Foods

Fill up! All the soup you can eat! All the vegetables you can eat! All the vegetable juices you can drink! You *can* diet without feeling starved. And you can eat all you want for very little money.

In order to make everyone's life as comfortable as possible and also in order to increase certain nutrients, the Choice Filler Foods offer two ways you can continue to eat as much as you want without adding significant calories that will put on additional weight. In fact, because of the specific electrolyte balance we are

High-Potassium Foods

Food	Amount	Potassium (mg)	Calcium (mg)	Magnesium (mg)	Vitamin C (mg)	Folacin (mcg)	Iron (mg)	Calories
asparagus, raw	4 spears	222	18	16	26	87	0.8	21
bamboo shoots, raw	1 cup	707	17	*	5	*	0.7	36
beet greens, cooked	1 cup	664	198	106	30	0.05	4	36
Brussels sprouts, cooked	1 cup	409	48	*	135	0.05	1.6	54
cabbage, cooked	1 cup	236	64	13	48	26	0.4	29
cauliflower, raw	1 cup	295	25	24	78	55	1	27
celery, cooked	1 cup	299	39	4	7	8	0.2	17
chard, cooked	1 cup	533	121	97	27	0.04	3	30
collards, cooked	1 cup	524	376	84	152	0.15	2	66
cucumber, raw	1 cup	160	17	10	11	15	0.3	14
endive, curly	3½ oz.	294	81	10	10	142	1.7	20
kale, boiled	1 cup	243	206	31	102	0.06	2	43
kohlrabi, raw	1 cup	554	61	55	98	0.015	0.75	43
lettuce, looseleaf	1 cup	174	45	10	12	24	0.92	12
mushrooms, raw	3½ oz.	375	13	7.7	3	0.016	1.4	35
mustard greens, cooked	1 cup	440	276	*	96	*	3.6	46
parsley, raw	3½ oz.	727	203	41	172	116	6	44
peppers, sweet green	3½ oz.	213	9	18	128	19	0.7	22
radishes	3½ oz.	322	30	15	26	24	4	17
spinach, cooked	1 cup	583	167	106	50	164	4	41
strawberries	1 cup	246	31	18	88	24	1	55
tomato juice	1 cup	454	14	8	32	52	2	38
vegetable juice	1 cup	442	24	*	18	32	1	34
watercress, raw	3½ oz.	282	157	20	79	0.017	2	19
zucchini	1 cup	282	50	21	18	0.04	0.8	24

* No value has been determined, but there is reason to believe that a measurable amount may be present.

after, i.e., a higher potassium intake, you are likely to lose weight as you shed excess fluids. (See Chapter 15 for more about the reasons for increasing your potassium intake.) *You should be aware that if you add salt to these foods, you can totally prevent such loss of fluids.* Many people, particularly women, retain excess fluids. Get rid of the salt and eat or drink as much of these foods as you want.

The High-Potassium Foods and the Basic High-Potassium Soup can be added to any of the diets at all, though people on the Raw Diet may choose to omit cooked soups and eat only raw soups, juices, and salads. Those on the Two-Minute Diet may choose to leave out the soup some days because of the time it takes to prepare. In that event, they should be sure to substitute some equally nourishing foods to meet daily requirements.

The High-Potassium Foods

Adding the foods listed in the table to your diet is easy and provides plenty of chewy, tasty fillers to prevent hunger and provide fiber and other nutrients. Use your imagination:

- Carry them to lunch as finger foods.
- Stir-fry them along with your other foods with a little dark sesame oil.
- Put them through a juicer for a really refreshing glass of vegetable juice (add spices if you like — no salt!).
- Steam them with a small amount of Low- or No-Calorie Salad Dressing (pages 245–247).
- Add them to stews.
- Make them into a salad.

Cooking concentrates these low-calorie, high-potassium foods, most of which are high in fiber, into smaller amounts — a salad bowl of spinach becomes a cup of cooked spinach, four stalks of celery become a glass of celery juice. Drink or save for use in soup any water you use in cooking or steaming, as that is where the potassium (and many other nutrients) will be concentrated.

Basic High-Potassium Soup

The Basic High-Potassium Soup is the foundation of the High-Nutrient Soup used in the Lean, Clean Machine Diet and also highly recommended as a regular part of each of the other diets in this book. There are a number of variations suggested here so you can choose the ones that fit your circumstances. The soup can be prepared with a base of water or Bone Stock (see below). The Bone Stock is necessary when using the soup to supplement the High-Protein, Low-Carbohydrate Diet in order to meet calcium requirements. You may want to use the bone soup base anyway because it tastes so good.

Basic High-Potassium Soup
1 bunch very green celery
1 pound green beans
1 pound zucchini
1 bunch parsley (about 1½ cups leaves)
1 cup chopped green onion (scallions)
Herbs (optional)
2 quarts distilled water or spring water

Clean the vegetables well under cold running water, then cut up into coarse chunks or fine pieces, as you prefer. Put the prepared vegetables, along with any herbs you choose, into 2 quarts simmering water (don't use city water — lengthy simmering concentrates unwanted chemicals) and simmer further for an hour or more.

This quantity provides the base for one day's serving of the High-Nutrient Soup called for in the Lean, Clean Machine Diet.

Read on for a number of ways to vary the soup.

High-Nutrient Soup. The high-nutrient version of the Basic High-Potassium Soup is described in detail with the Lean, Clean Machine Diet (Chapter 11). Using *half* the High-Nutrient Soup recipe daily to supplement any of the diets in this book completes virtually all nutrient requirements. Thus, your daily soup portion would consist of half the Basic High-Potassium Soup recipe augmented on a rotating basis by half the small amounts of liver, wheat germ, and oysters outlined in Chapter 11. You may in fact decide to consume a full soup portion every other day instead of half a portion each day. In this case, just be sure that over the course of the ten days the additions to the soup total at least ⅜ cup wheat germ, ⅛ pound liver, and 1½ oysters.

BASIC HIGH-POTASSIUM SOUP: NUTRIENT ANALYSIS

Here are the nutrient values of the Basic Soup without additions. As you can see, this simple vegetable concoction has a lot to offer on its own.

Vitamin A	14,000 IU	Magnesium	380 mg
Vitamin B-1	0.95 mg	Phosphorus	599 mg
Vitamin B-2	1.5 mg	Protein	25 gm
Vitamin B-3	11.2 mg	Zinc	15 mg
Vitamin B-6	1.8 mg		
Vitamin B-12	0	Calories	432
Vitamin C	436 mg	Carbohydrates	96 gm
Calcium	801 mg	Crude Fiber	12.8 gm
Vitamin D	*	Potassium	4528 mg
Vitamin E	7.6 IU	Fats (all)	2.1 gm
Folacin	608 mcg	Cholesterol	0
Iodine	*	Sodium	544 mg
Iron	13.5 mg	Sugar	0

Nutrient values calculated with Health-Aide nutrition software, Programming Technology Corporation, San Rafael, California, 1982.
* Values for vitamin D and iodine are indeterminate.

Filling and Nutritious Soup Variations. The High-Nutrient Soup is the best choice for filling unmet RDA requirements, as it is high in nutrition, high in roughage, and very filling. You can make it delicious by seasoning with freshly squeezed lemon juice and spices and herbs, if you wish. Instead of making soup, you can also steam the vegetables or eat them raw. Here are some ideas:

1. Eat the soup as is, leaving in the cut-up vegetables.
2. Purée the cooked soup (a little at a time) in the blender.
3. Strain the soup, squeezing out the vegetables well after straining, and use the broth. Add a few finely chopped onions or parsley for garnish. (Variations 3, 7, and 8 lack roughage but are quite delicious. If you wish to use these variations, make sure you have your roughage in the core diet.)

4. Add some foods from the core diet (grains, legumes, fish, poultry) to make a heartier soup or stew.

5. Steam the vegetables with a little water to the degree of doneness you desire. (Save even that little water for your next soup pot.)

6. Cut the fresh vegetables into a plastic bag to carry throughout the day. (Better for your teeth when they are fresh and crunchy.)

7. Put the fresh vegetables through a juicer and drink immediately. Or juice most of the vegetables and use for cold soup with the rest of the vegetables cut into small chunks. Water can be added if straight juices are too strong for your taste.

8. Vegetable juice can be made into a gelatin mold for summer or winter salad. Dissolve 1 tablespoon or envelope plain gelatin in warm water and add to 2 cups fresh juice. Add lemon juice to taste. Refrigerate for a few hours to set.

9. Make a raw soup by putting a few fresh vegetables at a time through a blender or food processor, using enough water to help the blending, till all are of soup consistency.

10. Little time to cook? Pressure-cook above mixture for 2 to 10 minutes.

11. Try freezing strained or unstrained *raw* broth or juice for a frozen soup sorbet (add lemon juice to taste). Stir often while freezing to keep smooth; gelatin can make consistency even smoother. Use a few finely chopped vegetables as a garnish.

Further Additions to the Soups. There are many ways to make good, nutritious soups that will keep your calorie count low and your stomach full, and will cost you next to nothing. Try adding these to either the Basic Soup or the High-Nutrient Soup for even greater appetite satisfaction; add what you need for you and your family:

- cornmeal, brown rice, wheat berries, rye berries, whole millet, whole barley
- black beans, kidney beans, lima beans, soybeans
- whole-grain noodles, rolled oats
- fish, shrimp, chicken, veal, beef, pork (shred fine for flavor, looks, texture)

Cooking time for these additions will vary from 3 hours for soybeans to just a few minutes for shrimp or chicken; consult your favorite cookbook. (Using a pressure cooker will reduce cooking times dramatically — even soybeans succumb in about 30 minutes.)

Garnish your soups to make them more beautiful and more delicious. Try these or any other garnish that appeals to you:

- chopped parsley, celery leaves, or scallions
- watercress
- thin slices of lemon or lime
- a little grated romano or Parmesan cheese
- chopped sweet red or green pepper (or both)
- fresh dill, basil, or other herbs
- caraway, sesame, or other seeds

Bone Stock

Bone Stock is a great base for the soups in this book. It adds flavor and nutrition to any soup. As mentioned elsewhere, this stock is especially important to those of you using the High-Protein, Low-Carbohydrate Diet, to help fulfill calcium requirements.

One of the cheapest ways to collect bones for your soups is to keep a plastic bag in the freezer and after every meal put all bones from chicken, fish, or meat immediately into the freezer bag. Another way is to ask your fish market to save you fish carcasses when they are filleting fish. They invariably throw them away if you don't take them. These carcasses are very good sources of calcium and other minerals and are not too bad a source of protein because of all the flesh and cartilage left on them. Other sources of bones, but which you generally have to pay for, are:

beef	lamb	chicken
veal	mutton	turkey
pork		

The bones from younger animals (veal, lamb, and fryers) are to be preferred because they have more cartilage than those from older or full-grown animals and will usually not have as much attached fat.

Bone Stock
2 pounds bones
2 quarts distilled water or spring water
(or enough to cover bones)
1 cup tomatoes *or* ½ cup vinegar
1 medium onion, halved (optional)

Combine all ingredients in a large stockpot, cover, and bring to a boil. Lower the heat and simmer 2–3 hours or more, with the pot lid barely askew to keep the soup from cooking too briskly; or pressure-cook 1 hour.

Strain the stock carefully to remove all bits of bone, then chill it to allow the fat to solidify on top so it can be easily removed. The broth is now ready to be used on its own or as the base for other soups.

Preparing and Cooking Bones
Bone Stock is exceedingly simple to prepare, but a certain amount of care does need to be taken in order to achieve optimal results.

The Bones. Chicken and turkey bones can be put into the cooking water as is. Other larger bones need to be split so that the center of the bone — the bone marrow — can be open to the water. The joints, which tend to be softer than the long bones, have calcium that is more easily available and have much protein-rich cartilage covering their surface. Bones from younger animals tend to make soups that will jell when cold. Larger and longer bones will need to be cut into pot-sized pieces. Few people can manage this at home. Your grocer usually has the tools for it, so ask him to cut them for you. A pound of bones for each quart of water is a good measure.

The Water. The usual city water is not to be used for soup. Though some chemicals used in keeping the water free of disease-bearing bacteria would be boiled away, others would be concentrated. I suggest you start with two quarts of distilled or spring water. Though the water must be brought to a boil after the bones have been added, there is no necessity to continue to boil the soup mixture. A simmer is fine and keeps the air nice and moist and smelling good in the winter. It does use more fuel of one kind or another to cook the soup this way, however, and it may prove to be too warm in the summer.

The Pot. An excellent and money-saving alternative for cooking soup, summer or winter, is to use a pressure cooker. The pressure cooker leaches much more calcium from the bones in much less time. A half hour will usually do the job of two to three hours in a regular soup pot.

The same acid that I suggest to dissolve the calcium in the bones will also dissolve your cooking pot to some extent. (That is why spaghetti sauce, if left to cook down in an aluminum pan, and tomato juice left in a can for a day or so, will begin to taste strange.) *I suggest that you never use an aluminum pot to cook even slightly acid foods!* A stainless steel pot does not tend to lose as much surface to the acid. You can buy both soup pots and pressure cookers in stainless steel. An enamel-lined pot is also a good choice.

Making the Calcium Available. The calcium in bones is deposited very securely. It will not dissolve in water alone. Some acid, such as that found in tomato or vinegar, must be added to the cooking water if you are going to leach the calcium from the bones into the soup. Add either a cup of tomatoes, or a half cup of any kind of vinegar to the water at the same time that you put the bones in. The smell and taste of the vinegar will disappear as the calcium is dissolved from the bones. Many people add an onion in with the bones, both for flavor and because it smells so delicious.

The smaller and lighter bones from most fish carcasses will become so soft after pressure-cooking that you can often put bones and all into a blender and have enormous amounts of calcium and protein for only the cost of some vinegar, the cooking, and the blending. You cannot find a cheaper source of these nutrients. And it makes a delicious, very rich, very thick soup stock.

Straining the Bone Stock. The nature of bones is that they tend to splinter as cooking continues. You must always strain bone soups to remove any tiny fragment of bone that may be left in the stock. This is an important step and must be taken *before* you add other foods such as vegetables to the stock.

More Useful Hints About Soup

You are perhaps starting to get the idea: The nutrient potential of the soups in this book is extremely high. Even if you try no other idea I've suggested, I hope you will give the soups a try (and for more than just a few days — changing our habits and our health takes time). Here are a few more ideas.

- You can add as little or almost as much water as you like as long as you continue to taste for flavor. If you add too much water, add a few more vegetables or some herbs.
- Soups are better the second or third day, so make plenty and keep them in your refrigerator or in your freezer. In this way you can always have something both inexpensive and delicious on hand for company.
- Soups tend to be good whether hot or cold, jellied, thick or thin.
- Even a low-calorie soup can be very filling.
- Soups are very easy to store, to eat, or to drink.
- Cold broth from the refrigerator is a lot more satisfying than water.
- The soups are designed to be high in potassium and will help you lose more water weight if that is the type of excess weight you carry.
- The soups are designed to be low in calories and will help you lose fat weight if that is the type of excess weight you carry.
- Soups are extremely advantageous for people in a hurry, people who need to stay feeling full, and older people who have difficulty chewing and swallowing with resulting problems in keeping their potassium level up so that they can continue to feel energetic.
- After soup has cooled, it is easy to skim almost every last bit of fat.
- Those who are allergic to dairy products will find the soups a delicious and low-calorie way to get all their daily requirements of calcium.
- I have purposely designed the soup to fill your daily requirement for liquids besides other nutritive requirements. If you just cannot drink that much, reduce the quantity of the fluids before you add the vegetables or cook the soup down further once it is made.

- If your doctor for any reason has denied you roughage, you can strain the soup and still end up with an excellent diet except for the lack of roughage.
- Using the same green vegetable ingredients as suggested, you can chop or put small amounts of vegetables at a time through your blender or food processor with Bone Stock or distilled water till all the vegetables are liquefied. Add a small wedge each of onion and lemon (with peel) and as many fresh or dried herbs as you want for flavor. Change ingredients around to suit yourself. Wonderful raw! Put daily leftovers into the next day's cooked soup.
- If you are adding any foods from the cabbage family, remember never to let the heat get above a simmer. Or to prevent the cooked cabbage smell, use the bone soup base. Protein seems to help keep the odor of cooked cabbage under some control.
- To thicken broths without adding many calories, add Irish moss in small amounts; it has lots of minerals and few calories and is an excellent thickener.
- You can freeze the broth in ice cube trays (flavor it well) and use it to cool summer soups or fresh vegetable juices, as is. You can freeze fresh basil or mint in the cubes for special effects, or you can put the cubes through a heavy-duty blender and serve the sherbet soup in dessert glasses on watercress with fresh herbs and lemon or lime slices for flavor and garnish. Use as an elegant appetizer.
- Heavily jelled soups can be served as is, again with beautiful garnishes, or can be molded. The jelled soups also look wonderful in glass with colorful garnishes.
- Soup or broth stocks, whether they are frozen or refrigerated, made from bones or vegetables, are more flavorful than plain water as a base for rice and any other whole grain, or for stews and casseroles.

More A-Rated Foods

On the following pages are many of the foods you should be adding to your daily diet to take the place of low-nutrient, high-calorie, overprocessed, overrefined, and overpriced packaged foods.

Fruits

Many people prefer to have several pieces of fresh fruit a day to fill their calorie requirements. Count calories *and* nutrients. (You will need a good source book to do this.) There are vegetables offering more vitamin A and vitamin C than any fruit, so look to the vegetables for best low-calorie nutrition.

Fresh Fruits

When a serving of fresh fruit is called for in one of the daily menu plans, select a fruit (or a serving size) that is under 100 calories. Choose a variety of fruits rather than eating the same ones day in and day out.

Food	Amount	Carbohydrates (gm)	Crude Fiber (gm)	Calories
apple	1 med.	24.0	1.8	96
apricot	3 avg.	13.7	0.7	55
banana	1 avg.	33.3	0.8	127
blackberries	1 cup	18.6	5.9	84
blueberries	1 cup	22.2	2.2	90
cantaloupe	¼ avg.	7.5	0.3	30
cherries	1 cup	20.4	0.52	82
grapefruit	½ med.	10.8	0.2	41
grapes	1 cup	26.0	0.9	107
guava	1 med.	15.0	5.6	62
honeydew	2" wedge	11.5	0.9	49
mango	1 fruit	28.8	2.7	152
nectarine	1 avg.	23.6	0.6	88
orange	1 avg.	16.0	0.9	64
papaya	½ med.	15.0	1.8	58
peach	1 med.	9.7	0.69	38
pear	1 avg.	30.6	2.8	122
pineapple	1 cup	21.2	0.5	81
plums	2 med.	17.8	0.4	66
raspberries	1 cup	16.7	4.0	70
strawberries	1 cup	12.6	2.0	56
tangerine	1 med.	10.0	0.5	39
watermelon	6" × 1½" piece	38.4	1.8	156

Nuts and Seeds

Nuts and seeds concentrate nutrients and are high in the unsaturated fatty acids that we need for the health of cells. They are an extremely valuable food group. Nuts and seeds are very high in calories (see page 264 for the fat content of some nuts and seeds), so eat only a few if the calories worry you. But they are an excellent food to include in your diet on a daily basis. Remember, roasting of these foods reduces digestibility, salting of nuts and seeds throws off the sodium-potassium balance, and rancidity destroys their usefulness. So try to buy them in small packages that can be used up quickly; eat them raw and very fresh; keep them refrigerated till use, or buy them in vacuum-packed cans (refrigerate after opening).

Nuts and Seeds

Buy the nuts and seeds you like in measured amounts, mix them together, and keep them in a jar in the refrigerator ready for use in meals or as snacks. The calorie amounts given here are for ¼ pound shelled nuts or seeds and will help you estimate the actual calorie count in your personal mix.

Food	Calories	Food	Calories
almonds	678	pili nuts	759
Brazil nuts	742	pine nuts	720
butternuts	713	pistachios	674
cashews	636	popcorn (unpopped)	438
chestnuts	220	safflower seeds	698
filberts	719	sesame seeds (whole)	639
hickory nuts	763	sunflower seeds	635
macadamia nuts	784	walnuts, black	712
pecans	779	walnuts, English	738

Foods High in Complex Carbohydrates

Once you have taken care of your nutrient needs, you may want to fill your calorie needs with foods high in complex carbohydrates. Whole cultures have risen and endured on such foods as rice, wheat, corn, millet, beans of every variety, and even potatoes, taro root, and all varieties of these. But these were active peoples, engaged in farming, cutting wood, fishing, hunting; and lots of calories were needed, far more than the average sedentary person of today can expend. There is not a single commonly known nutrient in these foods that you can't get, with fewer calories, from the recommended foods in the core diets. If you feel you cannot live without the filling effect you get from these foods, you can use a variety to fill your calorie needs healthily.

High-Carbohydrate Vegetables

Stay aware that the nightshade family, of which potatoes are a member, has been claimed by some to be associated with certain forms of joint pain. Also, potatoes and yams are higher in calories than the other foods listed.

Food	Amount	Carbo-hydrates (gm)	Crude Fiber (gm)	Potassium (mg)	Calories
Jerusalem artichoke, raw	4 sm.	16.7	0.8	*	42
parsnip, raw	½ lrg.	23.1	3.0	587	102
potato, baked	1 lrg.	32.8	1.2	782	145
rutabaga, cooked	1 cup	13.9	2.0	284	60
squash, winter, baked	1 cup	31.6	2.6	945	129
sweet potato, baked	1 avg.	37.0	1.8	342	161
turnip, cooked	1 cup	7.6	1.35	291	36
yam, baked in skin	1 cup	48.2	1.8	*	210

* No value has been determined, but there is reason to believe that a measurable amount may be present.

Breads, Muffins, Rolls, and Crackers

You may want complex carbohydrates in the form of breads, muffins, rolls, and crackers, but if you are or think you might be allergic to wheat, you would best have instead products made of rye, corn, or rice. I have purposely left out any white-flour products. Read labels to choose lowfat crackers and breads.

Food	Amount	Carbohydrates (gm)	Crude Fiber (gm)	Calories
Ak-mak crackers, whole wheat	2	9.4	*	59
muffin, bran	1 avg.	17.2	0.72	104

Food	Amount	Carbohydrates (gm)	Crude Fiber (gm)	Calories
muffin, whole wheat	1 avg.	20.9	0.6	103
pita, whole wheat	1 avg.	24.0	*	140
roll, whole wheat	1 avg.	18.3	0.6	90
toast, whole wheat	1 slice	11.0	0.4	55
cornbread	2" sq.	13.1	0.2	93
Ry-Krisp	2	9.6	0.3	42
tortilla, corn	6"	13.5	0.3	63
whole rice rounds	3"	7.6	*	35

* No value has been determined, but there is reason to believe that a measurable amount may be present.

Whole Grains

All grains may cause allergic reactions in sensitive individuals. Rice seems to give the fewest problems, so rice is listed by itself below the other grains. If you don't use prepared foods, you need never fear an allergic response to an ingredient you didn't know was there. Using a quite small amount of grains or legumes to which you are sensitive, and not using the same grain or legume twice in a row, can for many avert an allergic reaction. Keep track of what you do react to.

Food	Amount (dry)	Carbohydrates (gm)	Crude Fiber (gm)	Calories
barley	¼ cup	38.5	0.5	174
bran, oat		12.8	6.0	83
bran, wheat		8.8	1.3	30
buckwheat groats		30.0	4.0	137
bulgur		32.2	0.7	151
corn grits		30.0	0.15	145
cornmeal		2.2	0.3	107
millet		41.5	1.8	187
oats		13.75	0.25	78
rye berries		32.5	0.87	148
wheat berries		30.0	10.0	145
wheat germ, toasted		12.0	0.4	92
rice, brown		9.5	0.4	176

Legumes: Beans, Peas, Lentils

The quantities listed are appropriate for a single meal for one person. Cooking should be done in larger amounts to prevent burning and wasting of resources. Presoak the beans overnight, drain (use the soaking water to water your plants!), cover with water, bring to a boil, then simmer till done. Try mixing several legumes and grains, before or after cooking according to the effect you want, for new flavors and mixing of colors. Try them as appetizers, main courses, salads, soups. Plain legumes, like plain pasta, can be very boring. On the other hand, spiced and herbed legumes can be incredibly delicious.

Food	Amount (dry)	Carbohydrates (gm)	Crude Fiber (gm)	Calories
azuki beans	¼ cup	14.6	1.0	82
black beans		30.0	2.2	170
black-eyed peas		25.0	1.8	146
chickpeas		30.0	2.5	180
kidney beans, red		27.5	1.95	159
kidney beans, white		27.5	1.95	153
lentils		27.5	1.85	162
lima beans, white		30.0	1.9	155
navy beans		32.5	2.2	174
pinto beans		30.2	2.0	168
soybeans		17.5	2.5	212

Grain Cereals

Here are some ways to add fiber, nutrition, and appetite satisfaction to breakfast — or any other meal.

Basic Grain Cereal

Use ¼ cup (dry) of any of the grains in the Whole Grains list. Bring ½–¾ cup water (or water and milk) to a boil in a small saucepan. The amount of water will vary depending on the grain chosen; when in doubt, cook the grain in a double boiler so the mixture won't cook dry, or simply allow excess liquid to bubble away after the grain is tender. Add the grain (mix cornmeal with ¼ cup cold water first, then stir slowly into the boiling water) to the boiling water, stir, adjust heat, and simmer, covered, till done. Cooking time will vary from a few minutes for rolled oats to about 90 minutes for wheat berries.

GRAIN, NUT, AND SEED CEREAL

This has been a favorite mixture of mine for thirty years. There is always some in the refrigerator to eat out of hand or to use as cereal. The nutrient amounts shown in the chart are for 1 cup or 3½ ounces as noted. Peanuts should be roasted but unsalted; all other nuts, seeds, and grains should be raw; use toasted wheat germ. Always store nuts, seeds, and grains in the refrigerator. Leave the foods whole or chop them very coarsely just before eating to give yourself a good chewing workout. If you want or need to, you can put the ingredients through a blender a few at a time.

Serve the mixture preferably over plain yogurt or with milk (for more calcium). For variety, spoon fresh fruit or blackstrap molasses over the top.

Feel free to add or subtract any nuts or seeds that will make it more interesting or delicious for you (even cut up dried fruits such as apricots or prunes if you don't have a problem with them and can afford the calories on your particular diet).

A ¼ cup serving of this Grain, Nut, and Seed Cereal, not counting yogurt, fruit, or molasses, should amount to about 170 calories.

Food	Amount	Manganese (mg)	Potassium (mg)	Magnesium (mg)	Calcium (mg)	Iron (mg)	Phosphorus (mg)	Protein (gm)	Calories
wheat germ, toasted	3½ oz.	13	947	365	47	9	1084	25	391
wheat bran	3½ oz.	11	1121	598	119	15	1276	16	353
almonds	1 cup	3	1098	369	716	7	716	26	906
Brazil nuts	1 cup	4	1001	444	260	5	970	20	1001
hazelnuts	3½ oz.	6	350	56	44	1	232	7	380
peanuts, roasted	1 cup	2	97	252	602	3	577	37	842
pumpkin seeds	1 cup	*	*	*	71	16	1602	41	774
sunflower seeds	1 cup	2	1334	55	174	10	1214	33	812
sesame seeds, unhulled	1 cup	*	725	270	1160	10	616	19	582

* No value has been determined, but there is reason to believe that a measurable amount may be present.

Quick High-Fiber Cereal
Add ½ cup boiling water to a mixture of ¼ cup toasted wheat germ and ¼ cup oat bran. Stir to blend and allow to stand a few minutes till water is absorbed. This breakfast has about 175 calories and contains 6.4 grams of crude fiber. (Try this only if you have no wheat allergies.)

For Low Carbohydrates
The following lists contain the foods to be used with — or in place of — the High-Protein, Low-Carbohydrate Diet (Chapter 9). The foods in the following lists either totally lack or are very low in carbohydrates. They are useful for weight loss in those people who can feel good on a low-carbohydrate diet. Experiment. This type of diet is effective also for those who want extreme definition of muscle, such as body developers. The Basic High-Potassium Soup, because of its minimal fat content, will encourage you to metabolize your own stored fats.

No-Carbohydrate Foods
These foods have absolutely no carbohydrates. The seafood list includes no freshwater fish because of widespread pollution of lakes and rivers. In choosing meats, select Good grade rather than Choice or Prime beef for a lower fat, cholesterol, and calorie content. (Veal is even lower in these.) Young poultry with skin and visible fat removed will also be lower in fat, cholesterol, and calories than older, fatty birds.

The calorie counts given are for ¼ pound amounts.

Food	Calories	Food	Calories
Seafood		pollock	108
bluefish	133	salmon	246
cod	89	sardines, oil-packed,	
eel	264	drained	189
flounder	90	sea bass	118
haddock	90	shad	193
halibut	114	smelts	111
herring, Atlantic	200	snapper	106
herring, Pacific	111	swordfish	134
mackerel	180	tuna, water-packed	144

Food	Calories	Food	Calories
Beef		T-bone steak	161
chuck roast	292		
club steak	207	**Poultry**	
flank steak	158	chicken: backs	96
ground beef	203	breast	99
porterhouse steak	186	drumstick	78
rib roast	191	neck	82
round steak	153	thigh	109
rump roast	179	duck	303
sirloin steak	146	goose	293

Low-Carbohydrate Foods

Food	Amount	Carbohydrates (gm)	Calories
Fruits			
apricot	1 med.	4	18
blackberries	½ cup	9	42
cantaloupe	¼	8	30
fig, raw	1 fruit	10	40
gooseberries	½ cup	8	30
grapefruit	½ med.	13	41
nectarine	1 med.	24	88
orange	½ med.	10	32
peach	1 med.	10	38
pineapple	½ cup	9	41
strawberries	½ cup	6	28
tangerine	1 med.	10	39
Vegetables			
asparagus	4 lrg.	4	20
beans, green	1 cup	7	31
beans, wax	1 cup	6	28
beet greens	1 cup	5	26
broccoli	1 cup	7	40
Brussels sprouts	1 cup	10	56
cabbage, raw	1 cup	4	17
cabbage, Chinese	1 cup	3	18
cauliflower, raw	1 cup	5	27

Food	Amount	Carbohydrates (gm)	Calories
celery	1 cup	5	20
chard	1 cup	5	26
collards	1 cup	7	42
cucumber	1 cup	2	8
cress	1 cup	5	31
eggplant	1 cup	12	50
endive	1 cup	2	10
kale	1 cup	7	43
kohlrabi, cooked	1 cup	10	43
lettuce, iceberg	1 cup	2	10
mushrooms, raw	1 cup	3	20
mustard greens	1 cup	5	29
okra	1 cup	9	46
parsley	1 cup	5	26
peppers, sweet green	1 cup	4	18
peppers, sweet red	1 cup	7	31
radish, red	1 cup	8	4
scallions	1 cup	8	36
spinach, cooked	1 cup	6	41
spinach, raw	1 cup	2	14
squash, summer	1 cup	6	25
tofu	3½ oz.	2	72
tomato	1 med.	7	33
turnip	1 cup	8	36
turnip greens	1 cup	5	29
V-8 juice	1 cup	9	41

Low- or No-Calorie Salad Dressings

Here are ten extremely low-calorie salad dressings that really add flavor. The first nine average 3–4 calories a tablespoon. The tenth is a no-calorie dressing.

- My thanks to Charlotte Michaelson for this one!

    ½ envelope unflavored gelatin

    2 cups cider vinegar
    4–5 cloves garlic
    1 small onion
    2 tablespoons dried oregano
    1 tablespoon dry mustard
    3 tablespoons fresh basil or 2 tablespoons dried
    2 tablespoons dried dill weed
    1 tablespoon olive oil
    1 teaspoon ground cumin
    2–3 teaspoons honey (or to taste)

    ½ cup cider vinegar

Dissolve the gelatin by sifting it into ½ cup water and heating slowly as you continue to stir the mixture till it looks clear. Set aside.

Put the next ten ingredients in a blender and blend 3 minutes. Add the gelatin mixture and blend 2 minutes. Pour the mixture into a quart jar and add the ½ cup vinegar. Add water to fill the jar and cover tightly. This keeps for weeks in the refrigerator.

Experiment! Use less vinegar or try using lemon juice in place of vinegar. Use the herbs and spices you most prefer. Try Irish moss or pectin in place of the gelatin. Try peanut or safflower oil in place of olive oil.

- ¼ cup yogurt
    ¼ cup water
    ½ clove garlic, minced
    2 teaspoons fresh mint or dill, minced; *or* 1 teaspoon dried

- 1 tomato, mashed or chopped
  1 clove garlic, minced
  2 teaspoons fresh basil, minced, or 1 teaspoon dried
  ½ teaspoon olive oil
  ½ teaspoon lemon juice

- ½ cup yogurt
  1 cup grated cucumber
  1 teaspoon fresh dill, minced
  1 teaspoon fresh parsley, minced
  1 teaspoon scallions, minced

- ¼ cup yogurt
  ½ banana (or any other fruit), mashed
  Lemon juice to taste

- *Mix well, let sit overnight:*

  ¼ cup yogurt
  2 teaspoons grated Parmesan cheese (or any other cheese, crumbled)
  ½ teaspoon minced garlic or onion (optional)
  Caraway, curry, other herbs, spices (optional)

- 1 tomato, chopped
  1 scallion, minced
  ¼ cucumber, diced
  ½ inch piece hot pepper, finely minced
  ¼ teaspoon olive oil

- ½ cup yogurt
  ½ clove garlic, minced
  ½ teaspoon olive oil
  Fresh herbs, your choice

- *Great in place of mustard!*

  ½ cup yogurt or laban
  2 teaspoons horseradish

• *This is the no-calorie mix.*

Combine at least two hours ahead.
¼ cup water
1 clove garlic, minced
Few sprigs parsley, minced
Few basil leaves, minced

You can also create your own low-calorie dressing by thinning any standard dressing with water to an acceptable consistency. This works especially well with thick, creamy dressings. If your salad dressing is half water, you will be consuming half the calories you ordinarily would. Color and flavor your salad dressings with fruits, herbs, and spices. The more highly spiced and flavorful your salad is, the less dressing you'll tend to use and the fewer calories you'll consume. Save any leftover dressing in the refrigerator.

SEASONING

Make up several of the salad dressings, particularly the low- or no-calorie types, and keep them in your refrigerator. Use them to spice up fish, soups, or salads.

The spices will be much stronger for having had the water added to them.

Dying for Dessert?

Desserts can be delicious and yet low in calories. Be inventive. Make sherbet or tiny popsicles of crushed low-calorie fruit or fruits. Use a blender or food processor to crush the fruit. Put the fruit mixture into the freezer till half frozen, remove, and stir gently but thoroughly. If popsicles are wanted, put the partially frozen mixture into ice cube trays and insert sticks. For sherbet, any freezer-safe bowl with a wide top and a cover will do. Return the mixture to the freezer till firm. If sherbet is too firm when frozen, put it through the blender just before serving.

Here are a few suggestions for delightful frozen desserts:

- honeydew melon blended with a tiny bit of lime juice (try fresh mint leaves or a slice of lime on top if serving as sherbet)
- cantaloupe with very finely grated orange peel (if serving as sherbet, decorate top with orange slices)
- cantaloupe, watermelon, a small squeeze of lemon juice, and maybe two or three raspberries (not if you have to buy them special); use a few more raspberries for garnish
- strawberries with a little squeeze of lemon or lime juice and maybe a few raspberries for flavor
- grapefruit juice and pulp (without the segment lining and seeds); wonderfully refreshing between courses for special dinners
- orange juice and pulp (without the segment lining and seeds)
- pineapple with a little lemon or lime juice
- papaya with a squeeze of lemon
- mango with a squeeze of lemon
- peaches or apricots with a squeeze of lemon

You can make up all kinds of wonderful sherbets. Don't mix so many fruits together that the flavors get lost or overshadowed. A clean, clear taste suits this type of dessert. These unsweetened desserts are very refreshing.

Look for interesting small ice cube trays, popsicle molds, and dessert dishes both for eye appeal and to control the amounts that you or your family or friends consume.

Low-Calorie Beverages
In general we naturally drink or otherwise consume an adequate amount of fluids if we have them freely available. But we tend not to be aware of just how available fluids are in many of the foods we eat.

For instance, if you put one normal-sized rib of celery through a juicer you get back ¼ cup of fluids — water combined with vitamins and minerals. Even then you have not extracted all the water available from that stick of celery, or else dust would come out of the juicer and not soggy roughage. Fruits and vegetables can be as much as 95 percent water. Milk, cooked cereals, fish and shellfish can be over 85 percent water. Meat, poultry, cottage cheese, and eggs can be around 75 percent water. Cooked beans are almost 70 percent water. Even nuts and crackers have some fluid content, though it is small.

Most adults need two to three quarts of fluid per day. Try to guess roughly how many glasses of water you would get in your daily diet. Count those that come from the foods you eat and from the fluids you drink. A safe rule of thumb is to consume six to eight cups of fluids *as fluids* per day.

If you normally find taking plain water, tea, or coffee uncomfortable, or if you tend to hold fluids in your tissues (swollen eyes, swollen ankles and legs), try getting your fluids from the soup recipe recommended so highly in this book. This recipe will help you to lose excess fluids because of its high potassium-to-salt ratio. Do not add salt to your foods if you hold fluids in excess.

Here are some good ways to get the fluids you need without consuming sugar, caffeine, or other undesirable substances:

- Try a variety of herb teas. Though you may not like some, there are more and more arriving on the market. Some herbs can be toxic in large doses, so exercise caution, and don't drink only one kind of herb tea.
- A tablespoon or two of fresh lemon juice added to distilled or spring water is very refreshing. I even add a tablespoon or two of lemon juice to soups, beans, and fruits to give them a very fresh taste.
- The Bone Stock makes a wonderful hot drink winter or summer and is very low in calories yet high in calcium.
- The Basic High-Potassium Soup is also quite low in calories, and the strained broth is delicious as soup or beverage.
- Any of the foods from the High-Potassium list, when put through a juicer, make a wonderful fresh drink and are very rich in nutrients. When you first begin to use fresh vegetable and fruit juices, be sure to count your calories. Though these foods are low in calories, it can take several of them (four or five ribs of celery, for instance) to make a glass of juice. Dark green leafy vegetables must be used in very small amounts, as they come through the juicer surprisingly strong-flavored and dark-colored. Experiment with different combinations.

More Tips on
Making Your Food Better and Better

Eat many more small meals. The larger the meal, the more storage of excess calories as fat.

Eat more fresh raw foods. Nutrients are lost in storage and in cooking of foods.

Use more fresh fruit. Ease refined sugars out of your diet: jams, jellies, ice cream, soft drinks, etc., which contain mostly calories with few nutrients. Don't pay to have naturally included nutrients removed.

Use more whole grains. Ease out refined grain products such as spaghetti-type products and white-flour cakes, pies, pastries, breads, and rolls. Again, you want to preserve nutrients natural to the grains.

Use herbs and spices. Well-flavored foods help ease out highly flavored prepared foods, such as lunch meats, pickles, hot dogs, chips.

Read labels! Ease out, as far as possible, additives of all kinds. If foods spoil easily, don't depend on additives. Buy all foods fresh, in small amounts, keep them refrigerated, and use them soon. Meats, fish, poultry, vegetables, fruits, whole grains, nuts, seeds, and oils (if you are going to use oils) should all be kept refrigerated until use and leftovers returned to the refrigerator immediately afterward. None of these products should *ever* be kept on the pantry shelves unless vacuum-packed. Once the seal is broken, vacuum-packed foods must be refrigerated also.

Use a steamer. Steaming foods tends to use less water. Even so, the water will pick up nutrients from the food being steamed and should be saved for use in soups.

Use a pressure cooker for all dried beans, peas, and legumes and all bones for quick cooking. Even soybeans are done in twenty to thirty minutes, without presoaking, in the pressure cooker. Sometimes add bone broth and vegetables to the other ingredients in the pressure cooker for flavor. Add the vegetables later, for brighter colors and more separated tastes and textures, within the mix. This is also a good method for those who would otherwise not eat fresh vegetables.

Use a juicer if you want to consume fresh, raw vegetables in large amounts. Juicing removes roughage but allows you to consume much more of many nutrients than you would if the roughage remained. One bunch of carrots will make about one eight-ounce glass of juice. (Drinking too much carrot juice over an extended period of time, though, can turn your skin yellow, so use a variety of vegetables.) Do not let fresh juice stand except if you're freezing it or using it for molded salads. Breakdown in nutrients and flavor begins as soon as it becomes juice. Wash your juicer immediately for ease of cleaning and to prevent pitting and clogging of the machine. Make wonderful cold soups, cold drinks, molded salads, popsicles, vegetable or fruit sherbets for soups or desserts, with fresh, raw juice as the base.

Use a food processor to fix fresh salads often. Wonderful for adding vegetables to soups just before serving. Don't go too heavy on the onion or garlic, but anything else — everything else — goes in. Clean the machine immediately after use. The plastic bowl tends to pick up odors. Cut up the foods just before the meal they are to be used for, as vitamin C degenerates quickly at exposed surfaces.

Use a blender for fresh soups and drinks, fish chowder, clam stew, fruit frappes; the variations are endless.

To save space, you may be able to find a single piece of equipment that takes the place of the last three mentioned, combining one motor with three or more different attachments.

❧ 15 ❧

"Chuck 'Em" — and Good Riddance!

At the same time that you are putting more and more good foods into your daily diet, you should be trying to eliminate the X-rated foods, foods that are downright detrimental to your well-being. The following foods should be removed from your diet if you are trying to lose weight, trying to build or rebuild your nutritional health, or trying to save money:

- foods with added salt
- foods with added sugar
- refined grain and flour products
- foods high in fat or with added fat
- prepackaged foods or foods that have been stripped of nutrients

Eliminating these foods from your diet and replacing them with simple whole foods such as those described in Chapter 14 *may be all you need to do* to stay well-nourished and keep your weight where you want it.

If you tend to eat lots of the foods listed above, start with one category and try eliminating just one or two foods a week till you have finally excluded them all. If you are going to eat any of the X-rated foods, at least be aware of what you are doing. *Read labels!*

Use Less Salt to Improve
Your Weight and Health

For many of us, too much salt can be hazardous to health. Who among us by now is unaware that there seems to be a link between consuming too much salt and high blood pressure, which can result in potentially fatal kidney disease, heart disease, or stroke? Excessive sodium (a major constituent of salt) in the diet can have other consequences that are far less dramatic but still take a toll on human health. Certainly the presence of too much salt in the diet is a definite hindrance to a weight-loss program.

Adding salt to your food is not only potentially life-threatening, it is totally unnecessary, since all the sodium we normally need is naturally present in the foods we eat. Eliminating foods with added salt should be a high priority in your food strategy.

Sodium and Potassium in Body Fluids

Sodium, potassium, calcium, and magnesium are the four major metallic elements whose compounds make the sea salty. Our bones, like limestone and seashells, are composed of compounds of calcium and magnesium, which do not dissolve *easily* but are deposited and dissolved, deposited and dissolved steadily throughout our lives.

On the other hand, all of the compounds of sodium and potassium are so easily dissolved they are never deposited in our bodies but always stay in solution. In the sea, sodium is far more plentiful than potassium, but on land the situation is reversed. Away from the seashore, sodium becomes rarer and rarer in the soil. Land plants have little sodium in them but they are quite high in potassium.

So rare does sodium become inland that land animals, which need sodium, can't live easily in what may appear to be beautiful green fields. That is why herds of cattle and deer must find or be given salt licks, because by eating only vegetation, they get mainly potassium. Our word "salary" reflects the times when soldiers from the interior lands in Europe were paid off in salt as the most

ALTERNATIVES FOR
GETTING SALT OUT OF YOUR DIET

The kidneys are specifically built to retain sodium. Sodium is used over and over again by the body — and in a salt-sensitive person, the body will hold fluids for extended periods of time, according to how much salt you have taken in and how sensitive you are to it. If you are one of these unlucky people, you can follow certain routines to help keep your salt level low enough that you can be comfortable and have your weight under better control.

- Use more herbs and less salt to season foods.
- Begin taste-testing salt substitutes till you find one you like well enough to use. (Start with a potassium–sodium mix if you really feel you must have some added salt.) But, *do without added salt completely if you can.* Don't force it. If you're comfortable without it, good; if not, try more gradual methods.
- Don't put the salt shaker on the table.
- Don't add salt to foods as you cook.
- Read all labels for sodium content. Look for terms such as sodium chloride, salt, brine, MSG, soy sauce, miso, tamari.

precious and valuable stuff they could carry home. Even today, in the highlands of New Guinea, for instance, salt is treated as the most precious gift a visitor can bring.

Because potassium is so much more plentiful than sodium in their food, land animals have developed skins and kidneys that retain sodium in the body but allow potassium to pass through freely. This is true for any land animal with a backbone, from frog to man. Humans have kidneys that excrete potassium readily but reabsorb the sodium from the fluid to be excreted. Our kidneys salvage the sodium in our bodies and reuse it! The potassium is excreted on a regular basis. And in our sweat the ratio of potassium to sodium is higher than it is in the plasma of the blood. In our blood plasma and in the fluid that lies between the cells, there is twenty times as much sodium as potassium. But inside the cells, the opposite is true. Potassium is twenty times higher than sodium. This difference is important to maintain; a good fraction of the food we consume goes into keeping up that difference by pumping sodium out of cells and potassium into cells, especially in the nervous system and muscles. That is necessary since in the course of doing the work of the cells, potassium leaks out and sodium leaks in, and the pumps in the cell wall must work to restore the proper balance. This simplified version of the physiology involved helps explain why overconsumption of sodium has become a problem.

In our civilized society, sodium has become plentiful and cheap in the form of table salt; few tables, however poor the home, are without it. At the same time, through the processing of plant foods, such as refining grains or boiling vegetables and throwing the water away, we cut down on the potassium ordinarily available from plants.

Thus we need to keep eating good sources of potassium, but it's easy to overdo the sodium intake. (This is by no means an indication that you should take potassium *supplements* — that has its dangers, too. Get your potassium *naturally,* from food.)

Steer Clear of Added Sodium

The foods in which you find salt aren't always the expected ones — the salted nuts, chips, and snacks. Often salt has been added to a food totally unnecessarily. At one time, salt was needed as a preservative, but we no longer need it for that purpose. There are many common foods to which salt is added:

    many nuts
    most chips
    all canned vegetables, unless so-called dietetic
    most baby foods
    most cake mixes
    cured meats and fats, such as fatback, bacon, ham, and
        corned beef
    most baking powders
    most barbecue sauce, catsup, soy sauce, and mustard

most canned beans
practically all prepared meats (lunch meats)
most biscuit doughs
most prepared cereals
almost all cakes, breads, and crackers
most cookies and cookie mixes

"Most" is a marvelous and hope-filled word. Ten years ago there were few of the foods mentioned above about which you could have said "most." They *all* were prepared with excessive amounts of salt, and a person who questioned it was considered some kind of nut. There was much research available even then and simple, commonsense observation to support the theory that some people were having ongoing problems with too high a salt intake. At last there is much better labeling and a general trend toward lowering salt intake. Now you can find a great variety of foods labeled "salt-free" or "salt-reduced," from nuts to cheeses to sauces — *if you look for them.*

We may have to wait many years before it becomes a general trend among food packagers to allow us to add our own salt, as we may need or want it. We do not need to have decisions about what we eat made for us by total strangers. If we are *not* given the choice by some manufacturers, we can change to brands that allow us freedom of choice. And is it expecting too much to hope that the joke "If it's salt-free it costs more" will soon be relegated to the past?

Despite the progress of the past few years, at this time *reading labels for sodium content remains absolutely necessary.*

Sodium Needs: Normal Versus Individual

The recommended safe intake of *sodium* has been set at 1100 to 3300 milligrams, about the equivalent of 3 to 8 grams of *salt.* Some rather rare disease conditions require an additional salt intake for a few individuals. On the other hand, some of us on a "normal" intake of salt can suffer uncomfortable or even severe consequences, as if we were taking too much. Our problems can range from simple symptoms such as puffy fingers and puffy rings under our eyes to more serious symptoms such as gaining water weight or suffering from high blood pressure or Ménière's disease

Selected Foods High in Sodium

Read labels! Low-sodium varieties of these canned and packaged foods are usually available, though you may have to hunt for them.

Food	Amount	Sodium (mg)
bacon, Canadian	¼ lb.	2144
bacon, sliced	¼ lb.	771
beans, with pork	1 cup	1158
beans, without pork	1 cup	844
beans, yellow wax, canned	1 cup	819
beef, dried chipped	3 oz.	3660
bologna	¼ lb.	1474
chili, with beans	1 cup	1354
corned beef	¼ lb.	1474
corned beef, with potatoes	1 cup	1188
cottage cheese	1 cup	918
crab, canned	1 cup	1600
frankfurters	¼ lb.	1262
ham, cured	¼ lb.	854
lobster, canned	¼ lb.	339
pickle, dill	1 lrg.	1428
pickle, sour	1 lrg.	1353
pork, link sausage	¼ lb.	839
potatoes au gratin, with cheese	1 cup	1095
potatoes au gratin, without cheese	1 cup	870
salmon, canned	1 cup	851–1148
sauerkraut	1 cup	1755
sauerkraut juice	1 cup	1905
soups, canned (most)	1 cup	700–1800
soy sauce	1 TBSP	330

(constant ringing in the ears and possible dizziness or even vertigo), which at times can be directly attributed to an upset in the sodium–potassium balance causing retention of fluids in the inner ear.

If you are not made uncomfortable by a normal or higher salt intake, it may be all right for you, as an individual. If you have any doubt about whether you are salt sensitive, or if you have any medical problem that you feel may be related to your salt intake, changing your intake may make a difference and should be discussed with your doctor. If your doctor wants you to use salt, it will be for an important medical reason. Follow his advice!

Getting Rid of the Effects of a High-Salt Meal

You usually know it if you have a tendency to retain salt. If you think you may, weigh yourself before going out to a Chinese dinner. The next morning weigh yourself again. Normally you would weigh less in the morning. If you retain salt, you will weigh more in the morning after such a meal (sometimes several pounds more!). If you are female, premenstrual or menopausal, you may be even more prone to water weight gain from salt retention. It is better to avoid the problem of salt and the resultant fluid retention, but we are not perfect in our instantaneous decision-making, especially when food looks and smells delicious.

If you are salt sensitive and have indulged in a high-salt meal, it could take anywhere from one to three weeks to get rid of the excess salt and fluid if you do not do something about it. You can help yourself to a great extent by cutting back your salt intake and by consuming foods to raise your potassium level. This may help you to rid yourself of the excess salt and with it the excess fluids. Drink high-potassium fluids such as the Basic High-Potassium Soup (Chapter 14), fresh vegetable juices (celery in particular), canned unsalted vegetable or tomato juices, apricot nectar, and orange juice. And choose foods from the High-Potassium list (Chapter 14).

You can also try sweating out some of the excess sodium (as many in northern Europe do) in a steam bath, sauna, or hot bath — though not if you have high blood pressure or other medical problems. A certain amount of sodium will be carried off in the perspiration, and as you replace *needed* fluids by drinking salt-free beverages, the overall effect is to lower the concentration of sodium in your system. (Hot baths will leave you feeling a little weak if carried too far. In any case it is better to take hot baths in the evenings only, before bed. Start the bath with warm water and bring it gradually to hot, till you are perspiring. This method should be used for no more than a half hour a night. If dizziness occurs, the time spent in the tub is excessive.)

Regular aerobic exercise (brisk walking is fine) will usually help you sweat off some excess fluids. Of course, active aerobic exercise should be used for this purpose only if you are fit enough already.

Important Note!

Many older women who have problems with aging kidneys, which can no longer excrete fluids efficiently, will lower their salt intake to avoid becoming overloaded with fluids.

If you are a female and over forty, you must stay aware that a lowered salt intake can reduce stomach acidity, which can prevent production of a substance called the intrinsic factor. A reduction of the intrinsic factor in turn impedes the absorption of vitamin B-12. An inability to absorb sufficient B-12 afflicts fully half of women over the age of sixty! One out of every two women that you know over the age of sixty may have a B-12 deficiency! Many end up in nursing homes because of this problem.

The symptoms of B-12 deficiency are commonly seen among older women, such as digestive disorders, tingling hands and feet, unsteadiness, joint problems, moodiness, and other problems that you can find listed in Chapter 17. In many cases the cause of these ailments is not "getting old"; it is getting B-12 deficient.

We should be able to grow old in good health. The proper amount of salt for each of us as an individual is necessary to our health. We can, very often, take in more sodium with less fluid retention if we keep our potassium level high. The soup recipes in Chapter 14 are a good place to start.

Stay Away from Added Sugar

Sugar, like sodium, is a nutrient we don't need to add to our diet. Our bodies can extract all the sugar they need from fresh whole foods. Yet sugar — actually refined carbohydrates in the form of sucrose, corn syrup, honey, and molasses, to name a few — is the most widely used food additive in the country. The hazards of overconsumption of sugar can range from tooth decay to diabetes to overweight. Most insidious perhaps is the fact that sugar fills us up with "empty" calories, crowding out foods that supply essential vitamins, minerals, and other nutrients.

All of the diets in this book are very low in added sugar because they are low in refined and processed food products. If you think you might not like a diet low in starches and sugars, take a look at the Sweet Diet (Chapter 4); it can get you off to a good start in terms of adding nutrient-rich and sweet-tasting carbohydrates to your diet. In the meantime, you should be trying to increase your sugar awareness. Even people who don't like "sweets" may be consuming much more sugar than they realize. Here are some common foods high in added sugar:

> soft drinks
> juice drinks (label must say "no sugar added"; "unsweetened"
>   allows manufacturer to bring sugar to level of previous
>   batches)
> jams, jellies, preserves
> peanut butter
> baked goods: cakes, cookies, pastries, pies, breads, many
>   breakfast cereals
> alcoholic beverages
> candies
> canned fruits in light or heavy syrup
> canned yams
> dried fruits
> mustard, catsup
> mayonnaise, salad dressings
> chutneys, pickles
> spaghetti sauce
> cured meats

We have a lot of help from health food stores and manufacturers now. Many of these products can be found with no sugar added. Use foods that are sweetened with added fruit juice only. Even in health food stores, *read labels!*

Toss Out Refined Grain Products

Improve your health and some of your problems with excess weight. Get rid of all white-flour products, those with the germ and the bran removed. *Read labels!* "Wheat flour" and "enriched wheat flour" printed on labels do *not* mean "whole wheat flour." "Corn flour" and "enriched corn flour" do not mean "whole-grain cornmeal." "White rice" or "enriched rice" does not mean "natural brown rice." Check the labels carefully. Whole wheat flour, whole cornmeal, and natural brown rice give you the roughage, vitamin E, potassium, magnesium, and calcium that come naturally in the whole grain (perhaps along with nutrients that we have yet to discover).

Why buy refined foods and then pay extra for supplements? Check the labels on all these foods in the store. Get your money's worth. Every one of these products is available in whole grain or whole-grain flour in today's market (mostly in health food stores and better supermarkets at this time). Keep asking till your grocer will stock whole-grain foods, or mail-order them if you must. Don't eat less than the best. Read labels constantly, especially when buying

breads	stuffing	pies
breading	cakes	puddings
breadsticks	cookies	pasta products
crackers	cupcakes	thickened gravies
croutons	muffins	
rolls	pastries	

Say Good-by to High-Fat Foods

We have, as a nation, serious problems with too high an intake of fat. When the facts are laid out simply, it is easy to see in which foods the percentage of fats and saturated fats is just too high. It has been suggested to us that dietary fats should represent no more than 30 percent of our daily calorie intake, with saturated fats accounting for no more than 10 percent of daily calories. Yet from one serving of meat and a salad with dressing we could easily be consuming 75 percent of our calories in fat!

Few of the people who come to me for nutritional advice consume less than 50 percent of their calories in fat. Check your own level for just a few days. You need to know. Most people are horrified at the results.

Fat Content of Selected Foods

The table shows you the proportion of fat and saturated fat in some common foods. More than 80 percent of the calories in bologna, for example, come from fats, and 35 percent of the calories come from saturated fats. Skinless chicken breast, on the other hand, gets only 18 percent of its calories from fat, and just 5 percent are from saturated fats.

Food	Calories in 3½ oz.	Total Fat Content		Saturated Fat Content	
		Calories in Total Fats	As % of Total Calories	Calories in Sat. Fats	As % of Total Calories
Lunch Meats					
bologna	304	248	81%	107	35%
ham/pork loaf	294	224	76%	96	33%
salami	311	230	74%	78	25%
Beef					
sirloin steak, broiled	387	288	74%	120	31%
chuck, pot roast	289	173	60%	72	25%
ground chuck, cooked	327	215	66%	72	22%
ground round, cooked	261	139	53%	57	22%
liver, fried	229	95	42%	26	11%
Pork					
chops, loin	391	285	73%	102	26%
ham, cured, roasted	289	199	69%	70	24%
bacon, cooked	611	468	77%	153	25%
Canadian bacon, cooked	277	158	57%	53	19%
Lamb					
leg, roasted	186	63	34%	36	19%
rib chop, broiled	407	320	79%	151	37%
Veal					
cutlet, broiled	216	100	46%	42	20%
loin chop, cooked	234	121	52%	51	22%

Food	Calories in 3½ oz.	Total Fat Content		Saturated Fat Content	
		Calories in Total Fats	As % of Total Calories	Calories in Sat. Fats	As % of Total Calories
Chicken					
white meat, no skin	166	31	18%	9	5%
dark meat, no skin	176	57	32%	24	14%
skin, fried in fat	419	260	62%	81	19%
Dairy					
buttermilk	40	8	20%	5	14%
milk, 3% fat	61	30	49%	5	14%
milk, 1% fat	42	10	24%	6	15%
cheddar cheese	403	298	74%	190	47%
cottage cheese, 2%	90	17	19%	11	12%
cottage cheese, 1%	72	9	13%	5	8%

Though the fats in fish are still to be counted in calories, the constituents of the fish fats will help keep your cholesterol level down.

Food	Calories in 3½ oz.	Total Fat Content		Saturated Fat Content	
		Calories in Total Fats	As % of Total Calories	Calories in Sat. Fats	As % of Total Calories
Fish					
cod, cooked	129	6	5%	0.9	1%
flounder, cooked	140	12	8%	3	2%
haddock, cooked	90	6	7%	0.9	1%
herring, canned	208	122	60%	23	11%
salmon, broiled	182	67	37%	12	6%
salmon, oil-packed, drained	141	53	38%	14	10%
tuna, oil-packed, drained	197	74	37%	27	14%

All of the foods listed on the previous pages contain cholesterol. In many countries these foods are used in small amounts for flavoring. There is no cholesterol in vegetables, nuts, seeds, grains, legumes, and fruits. It has been known for some time that vegetarians have much less heart disease than meat eaters, especially when they use no dairy products.

It must be acknowledged that nuts do have a high fat content and so must be eaten in small quantities.

Food	Calories in 3½ oz.	Total Fat Content		Saturated Fat Content	
		Calories in Total Fats	As % of Total Calories	Calories in Sat. Fats	As % of Total Calories
Nuts					
almonds	598	488	82%	39	6%
Brazil nuts	654	602	92%	157	24%
peanuts, roasted	585	448	77%	86	15%
sunflower seeds	560	426	76%	54	10%

No Fake Food If You Can Prevent It!

Even though you do your best to buy fresh, whole, nutritious foods, there are always going to be some problems. A major problem, to my mind, is additives. All are added, of course, on the supposition that food will be improved in quantity, looks, texture, color, or keeping qualities. Many things are added to and taken from your food during the growth period, the packaging period, the storage period, and the transportation period. Many of them you might rather do without — and certainly never meant to pay for.

A steadily growing number of people are trying to get foods as unadulterated as possible. Simple, clean, fresh, nutritious foods. How and what we are eating is coming under ever more serious scrutiny and consideration. Not just mothers who care about their baby's or entire family's health but single people who realize their largest responsibility in their own health care comes under prevention. Some people in desperation have taken to farming. That involves a serious change of lifestyle — and they still have to contend with polluted air and water, and the sprays from neighbors' farms.

Most people do not want to spend their whole life supporting this kind of lifestyle. To design a truly successful food strategy, you do not have to go to this extreme. But you do have to ask yourself, How far am I willing to go? There are going to be problems to deal with no matter how much of a purist you are. If it is only a matter of changing your buying and eating habits, the way is reasonably simple, since many of the better, or less tampered with, products are becoming more commonly available. But vigilance is the key to finding these products.

Two *"Convenience Foods"* You're Better Off Without

Bottled Salad Dressings. What could be more healthful than a nice fresh salad? Many dieters deceive themselves by topping that salad with "just a little" dressing. Two to three tablespoons of the usual bottled salad dressings amounts to more calories than those in a full bowl of salad greens. Most of those calories come from fats and oils. Some oil is *absolutely essential* for production of cell membrane and for other important functions. But we get enough fats and oils from foods such as poultry, fish, whole grains, and in particular, nuts and seeds. We have no need for any additional supply and will use it mainly for getting fatter (if not damaging our systems). Most bottled dressings are also laced with sugar, salt, and other additives — read the labels and see for yourself.

The thicker a salad dressing is, the more it clings to your food and the more calories you get from it. If you won't give up these convenience dressings, at least thin them down. You can cut in half the calories you use in salad dressing by mixing 1 tablespoon of dressing with 1 tablespoon water, vegetable broth, No-Calorie Salad Dressing, vinegar, or lemon juice. Mix the fluid in gradually for a smooth dressing, and if it takes a little less or a little more to make the consistency or the taste just right, you're in charge, you judge. For example:

2 tablespoons blue cheese dressing = 143 calories
1 tablespoon *each* blue cheese dressing and water = 72
    calories

2 tablespoons Italian dressing = 157 calories
1 tablespoon *each* Italian dressing and water = 79 calories

2 tablespoons mayonnaise = 204 calories
1 tablespoon *each* mayonnaise and water = 102 calories

2 tablespoons Russian dressing = 140 calories
1 tablespoon *each* Russian dressing and water = 70 calories

2 tablespoons Thousand Island dressing = 143 calories
1 tablespoon *each* Thousand Island dressing and water = 72
    calories

Even these low-calorie versions of familiar salad dressings supply fats and oils far beyond the needs of most of us. Try out the
Low- or No-Calorie Salad Dressings in Chapter 14, or try to use
less and less dressing each day. If you toss the salad longer to
spread the dressing around, less dressing doesn't taste like less.
The familiar flavor of our favorite dressings will sometimes divert
our attention completely from the slight difference made by thinning them.

Lunch Meats. If you're serious about dieting or improving the
quality of your foods, lunch meats should be high on your "chuck
'em" list. All of the lunch meats or prepared meats mentioned
below have

- protein and B vitamins, but you can get these from less expensive fresh meats
- many extra calories from the mixed-in added fat, which you
  can to some extent trim off fresh meats
- extra calories from starchy fillers, not found in fresh meats
- preservatives, which are there by law but are unnecessary in
  fresh meats
- generally a high salt content, not found in fresh meats

Some companies are now producing fat- and salt-reduced foods.
In general, even these improved prepared meats still cost much
more for a less nutritious product with preservatives added. *Read
labels!*

Calorie Content of Lunch Meats

The calorie counts listed below are for ¼ pound quantities. Compare them with those of fresh meats and poultry (¼ pound of cooked lean beef is about 170 calories, pork about 280 calories, chicken breast about 100 calories).

Food	Calories	Food	Calories
blood pudding	447	meat loaf	227
boiled ham	266	minced ham	259
bologna	345	mortadela	358
braunschweiger	362	polish sausage	345
brockwurst	300	pork and beef, minced	381
brown-and-serve sausage	446	pork sausage	565
capacola	566	potted meat	282
cervalati	512	salami	510
country sausage	392	scrapple	244
deviled ham	398	spiced pork	344
frankfurters	254–351	souse (little fat here)	208
head cheese	304	thuringer	349
knockwurst	316	vienna sausage	273
liverwurst	349–362		

Another Reason to Eat Whole Foods

Your entire digestive system is set up to do its various jobs in a very old-fashioned way. Chewing is meant to begin the breakdown of food and to expose more of its surface to digestion by breaking it into much smaller particles. Teeth, gums, saliva, taste buds, jawbone are all important parts of the digestive system. When we send food that does not need chewing to our stomach, it leaves our teeth, gums, even our jawbone in terrible condition. There is no tension to strengthen muscle and bone, and no pressure to force blood into and out of the gums to keep them healthy. We lose our teeth partly because of this. When we lose our natural teeth, our whole face sags and the jawbone, which no longer has teeth to support, generally will shrink at least a little. False teeth do only a third of the work that our natural teeth can do.

Crunchy or chewy unrefined or raw foods need to be kept longer in the mouth to prepare them for swallowing. Each new mashing of the food that you create by chewing releases more flavor. Crunchy, interesting foods that help keep our teeth and gums healthy go a long way toward providing satisfaction. When you eat a meal, the feelings of satisfaction, both in taste and fullness, lag about twenty minutes behind the time you start eating. Eating foods that require chewing for an extended period of time *might* cause you to eat less. You should begin to feel full while you are still trying to chew up crunchy foods thoroughly. It might be worthwhile to choose foods that will encourage a lot of chewing, not only to strengthen teeth and gums but also to satisfy your appetite with fewer calories. Serve them before meals or as an appetizer for best results. Terrific for television snacks.

 Cut fat, salt, calories, and preservatives! Read labels! Buy fresh meats—cheaper, more nutritious, less fattening!

The roughage in your food also helps control your weight as the digestive system burns calories trying to break down the fiber.

Mashing, juicing, and refining foods lowers or does away completely with the need to chew. Soft foods that slip down without needing to be chewed are barely tasted and leave you wanting more. More food, more taste, and so you will tend to eat more of refined foods. Unless you have so-called false teeth, try to avoid foods that don't need to be chewed. Watch out for deceitful foods — those that have crunch but no roughage, such as chips and crackers made from refined grains. They are crispy on the outside and may help your teeth and gums some, but they will clog you up inside. Too many refined, soft, and juiced foods will help cause you to lose your teeth and your regularity.

Eat Better Foods and Save Money

When you begin to read labels on a regular basis, you find that prepared foods for the most part are made up of refined foods (foods that have had their vitamins and minerals stripped) with salt added, with sugar added, with fat added, plus lots of additives that processors use to lengthen shelf life, make the foods appear fresher, improve their color and texture. In fact, the processors even add air and water, for which they charge us!

The food companies charge us most for the packaging! No one minds paying for a food that has been improved by having nutrients concentrated, such as wheat germ; or by vacuum-packing a food that would otherwise become rancid, such as oils; or by bottling (rather than canning) a fruit that will otherwise rot before it reaches the marketplace, such as peaches or apricots. We need to demand from the processors that they *improve* our diets by their processing, rather than treat us like a bunch of idiots who will pay for and eat anything as long as the picture on the package is pretty enough.

 Read labels! Eat unrefined foods! Keep chewing!

We don't have to put up with this. Take away the package, leave the vitamins, minerals, and roughage as they were, leave out the salt, sugar, fat, and other additives, and things are right where they started — fresh foods with vitamins and minerals still in place. The cost is cut by half or even more and there's much less trash to deal with. We can save half or more of our food money by preparing meals from scratch and we'll be healthier for it.

Simple foods are usually safe foods.
Simple foods are conservative foods.
Simple foods are usually the most healthful foods.
Simple foods are the cheapest foods.

If you are used to eating many prepackaged foods, with or without reading labels, you can improve your health in an almost startling fashion by deciding never to touch another refined, canned, frozen, or prepared food. And you'll save money.

❧ PART V ❧

Diet Master

❧ 16 ❧

Making It Work:
Designing Your Food Strategy

If you're embarking on a weight-loss program, there may be times when you stop losing weight, really come to a complete stop. And — horror of horrors — sometimes you'll even regain a few pounds! This is the time that you'll get a terrible temptation to quit trying. After all, if your body is going to let you down, what's the use?

Your body does not work on a daily schedule in all matters. Some of its systems operate in terms of fractions of seconds, some in terms of minutes and hours, some in days and weeks, some in months, some in years, and some (such as the aging process) over the whole lifetime. Losing and gaining materials in the body is balanced by a delicate and continuous, overlapping and intricate network of systems that are constantly readjusting at different tempos.

Plateaus and Other Problems

If you are working at eating well, you want your body to *show* you daily success, but it won't always do so. Look more closely and look differently. In the first place, recognize that changing systems take some time to reach a new equilibrium. Expect a few ups and downs for a while. Second, be aware that a lot of the systems that you do not watch may be getting better:

Your breathing may be improving.
Your arches may be rising.
Your circulatory system is having its load reduced.
Your back may not be so strained.

Your entire body is undergoing changes for the better! Don't look only for the pounds dropping away on the scale. Many of us have fallen off one diet after another because of this shortsightedness. You can choose to change to an alternative diet, or you can content yourself with slower weight loss if you like the diet you're on very much. Don't worry if your scale says you're not losing. As long as your output column remains higher than your input column, you will slowly and steadily make a turnaround.

If you mess up by eating the wrong foods at a meal, try to accommodate immediately by adjusting the rest of that day's calories and nutrients. You may someday stray from your eating plan for longer than a meal, even longer than a day. Try again! You must practice to become good at anything. Mistakes while practicing do not mean you're not going to succeed. You only fail if you quit trying!

Help When You're in Trouble

About to binge? Under stress? Ravenous? If, while you're learning self-control in diet, your stomach continues to scream for mercy, try sipping four to six ounces of hot or cold (whichever you find more satisfying) vegetable stock every half hour, or oftener if necessary. Keep a big bowl of fresh vegetables prepared and handy. Use as much as you want of the low-calorie salad dressings.

Remember that when you're under stress it is comforting to fall back into old habits, whether they happen to be good or bad. Resist the bad eating habits! Make it easy for yourself. Keep the right foods in your house or office. Prepare them ahead of time. Make them look as attractive as possible. Keep prepared soups and broths in the freezer and refrigerator, or on the stove or office hot plate. Keep the wrong foods out of reach (out of your house and office), out of sight, out of mind! Spice the soup heavily, if you choose. Throw some bright crunchy vegetables in at the last minute, if you choose. Keep your stomach feeling full! Keep your mouth busy if you need to! Give yourself every possible chance to succeed.

For Lowest Calories

If you are trying to lose weight and want to make some changes in your eating plan, you could choose foods from the following lists, which contain foods you can eat reasonably freely. As you are developing the best food strategy for you, these are the lowest-calorie foods available.

Foods with Only 18 to 50 Calories in a Full Half Pound

Food	Calories	Food	Calories
Seafood		kohlrabi	48
clams, in shell	31–36	lettuce, all	22–28
		mustard greens	46
Vegetables		peppers, sweet green	41
bamboo shoots	18	pumpkin, raw	42
beans, green	37	purslane	48
beans, yellow	34	radishes, all	34
beet greens	31	spinach	50
cabbage, Chinese	31	spinach, mustard	50
cabbage, green	49	spinach, New Zealand	43
cabbage, pak choy	35	watercress	40
cabbage, Savoy	49		
cauliflower	50	**Fruits**	
celery	29	cantaloupe	34
chicory greens	37	grapefruit	43
cucumbers	33	lemon juice	50
cucumbers, pared	23	lemons, peeled	41
dock	45	melon, casaba	31
eggplant	46	melon, honeydew	47
endive	31	watermelon	27

Foods with Only 51 to 80 Calories in a Full Half Pound

Food	Calories	Food	Calories
Vegetables		**Fruits**	
asparagus	55	jackfruit	62
beets	73	limes	54
broccoli	64	longans	74
cabbage, red	64	papaya	60
carrots	78	peaches, raw	71
celeriac	78	pineapple, raw	62
chayote	52	plums, greengage	72
chives	64	pomegranates	80
collard greens	73	tangelos	52
kale	73	tangerines	77
leeks	62		
mung beans, sprouted	80	**Grains**	
mushrooms	52–62	soybean milk	75
peppers, hot chili	57		
pumpkin, cooked	75		
turnip greens	52		

Foods with Only 81 to 150 Calories in a Full Half Pound

Food	Calories	Food	Calories
Seafood		**Vegetables**	
oysters, eastern	150	Brussels sprouts	94
smelts	122	corn, on cob	122
weakfish	132	dandelion greens	102
		lambsquarters	98
Dairy Products		okra, frozen	89
buttermilk	82	parsley	100
milk, skim	82	parsnips	147
milk, part skim	134	pea pods	114
yogurt, part skim	114	peas, carrots, frozen	125
yogurt, whole milk	141	potatoes	140
		rutabagas	89
		soybean sprouts	105

Foods with Only 81 to 150 Calories in a Full Half Pound

Food	Calories	Food	Calories
Fruits		granadilla	106
apples	93–123	grape juice	150
applesauce, unsweetened	93	grapes, American	89–99
apricots	109	grapes, European	135
apricots, water-packed	86	guavas	137
apricot nectar	130	mangos	101
bananas	131	nectarines	134
blackberries	91–125	oranges, whole	81–90
blueberries	89–127	peach nectar	109
boysenberries	82	pears	126
cherries, sweet	143	persimmons	143–147
currants	110–120	plums, damson	136
fruit salad, water-packed	134	raspberries, black	161
gooseberries	89	strawberries	81

Foods with Only 151 to 230 Calories in a Full Half Pound

Food	Calories	Food	Calories
Seafood		mussels	216
bullhead	191	octopus	166
burbot	186	perch, Atlantic	200
cod	177	pollock	216
crab	211	snapper, any	211
crab, canned	229	sandabs	179
crappy	179	sauger	191
crayfish	164	scallops	184
croaker	218	sea bass	218
cusk	170	shrimp	207
redfish	182	snails	204
flounder	179	squid	191
sole	179	sturgeon	213
grouper	198	tautog	202
haddock	179	tile	179
hake	168	tomcod, Atlantic	175
lobster	207		

Foods with Only 151 to 230 Calories in a Full Half Pound

Food	Calories	Food	Calories
Poultry		**Vegetables**	
chicken, young:		breadfruit	180
back	193	corn, off cob	188
breast	197	sweet potatoes	210
drumstick	157	yams	197
neck	165		
thigh	218	**Fruits**	
wing	163	figs, raw	182
turkey, young	202	plantain	195
(double calories for old birds)			
		Grains and Nuts	
Dairy Products		butternuts, in shell	200
cottage cheese,		soy curd (tofu)	164
uncreamed	195		

Premenstrual Weight Gain

Men who are dieting can usually come straight down in weight with no problem as long as they stick to their weight-loss diets. Many women will come down, hit a plateau, come down, hit a plateau. It can be very discouraging.

As women gain weight, the skin and muscles of their bellies will sag more and more, and stretch further and further. When women haven't got their weight under control, they tend to gain three to six, and even ten pounds and more, premenstrually, so that every time they are about to have a menstrual period, their bellies bloat and bulge. It is unsightly, and it is uncomfortable.

When dieting to lose weight, this type of woman before each menstrual period will tend either to hit a plateau — stop losing weight — or may even go up in weight, sometimes significantly. For some the extra weight comes off very quickly after each period. For others each menstrual period means a few extra ounces, which add up month by month, year by year, pregnancy by pregnancy, even on into menopause. A horrible and remorseless intrusion into their lives.

A great number of women who take hormones, either as a contraceptive or during menopause, will find it causes them to hold extra fluids. If you think that this may be the case with you, talk it over with your doctor. A smaller dosage or a change in medication might do away with the problem.

A diet that is low in salt and high in magnesium- and potassium-rich foods, on a daily basis, does help prevent water retention, helps you to rid your body of excess fluids, and so helps prevent a gain in water weight. Physical activity can also be a great help at such a time if your excess weight is not too exaggerated. A workout ambitious enough to cause you to perspire, exercise that you enjoy doing, that can be continued on a daily basis, can help you lose a lot of those fluids.

A Good Meal Is Made of Many Things (Mozart, Paper Plates, and an Executive Armchair)

There are many ways to enhance your enjoyment of food. Making mealtimes a relaxed, pleasant occasion will do much toward helping you stick with your good new habits.

- frequent small meals, for good absorption
- attractive surroundings — a window to look out or a beautiful corner
- a comfortable chair to lean back and relax in
- happy surroundings — politeness and manners do count
- maybe quiet music or stories read to you on tape
- nourishing foods attractively served
- good-smelling foods, fragrant with spices and herbs
- good-tasting foods, bitter to sweet
- good-textured foods, crunchy to smooth
- varying temperatures, hot and cold foods
- low-calorie, fresh foods, to fill you up
- a leisurely pace — having several courses extends the pleasure

If you have grown to hate washing dishes, try, as I once did, using paper plates and cups for a period of time. (To make up for the trees I so poorly used, I discontinued reading the daily newspaper. I don't mind knowing about matters that I can do something about. But to know of disasters makes me feel impotent and sad.) My meals became doubly delightful. There was no washing up, no putting away, no arguing with my mealmates, and no bad news. If we could use edible plates, maybe of pita bread or tortillas, we could do away with the trash as well.

Spices and herbs added to foods quite often will make your mouth water. Salivating is good for cleaning your teeth, keeping mucous membranes healthy, and adds amylase, one of the enzymes that begin the breakdown of carbohydrates. This saliva helps to moisten food as you chew and helps to distribute all those good flavors as well as make the nutrients more accessible for absorption. Herbs and spices can make you want to chew more just for the pure pleasure of it.

Foods with added herbs and spices tend to satisfy your hunger more easily. No matter what your age or what habits you've gotten into, you can enjoy your food more, keep your teeth cleaner, keep your gums healthier, keep your facial muscles stronger if you chew more because you like the flavor of the food more. Hot foods such as peppers of various sorts, if used in small amounts to begin with, can add a great deal of pleasure to an otherwise boring meal (be cautious!).

There are many different directions to go in flavoring foods, lots of different ethnic cooking, varieties of hot foods, bitter foods, sweet foods, sour foods. If you've gotten out of the habit of using spices and herbs, consider dipping into your cookbooks again, or try some of the exotic new ones on the market. Photographs in cookbooks alone should be enough to inspire you. Be careful to add to these recipes your own new know-how from this book, keeping fats, salt, sugar, and refined foods to a minimum. Some of the recipes will taste better for the changes. All of them will be better for your health.

Think You Need Supplements?

The best way to improve your nutrition is by increasing the nutrients in your food — by changing your diet. You can improve your diet without adding calories or bulk. There are several ways to do this. You can choose foods that naturally concentrate nutrients, as we have done in the Shine Diet. You can make your own fresh juices from fruits and vegetables. Juice maintains the freshness of raw foods, concentrates vitamins and minerals, and eliminates enormous amounts of bulk. A bunch of carrots will reduce to a single glass of juice. This juice is extremely easy for almost anyone to digest. It is especially good for those with digestive problems. Fresh juices should be consumed quickly, as standing for a period of time renders them less tasty. Using the soup recipes in this book as a starting point, you can add only high-nutrient foods to develop a low-calorie, nutrient-rich soup that will be delicious. Search out the best foods from the lists in this book. In most cases these options will help you to meet the nutritional demands of your body.

Only if you can't meet your needs in this way, or if you are just too busy to put in the extra time, should you consider the usually more costly avenue of regular supplements in the form of single vitamins and minerals, in various potencies, in pill, powder, or liquid form. If you have never studied nutrition as an aspect of your diet, then maybe a nutritionist and your doctor can tell you whether supplements are indicated for you in any case. Since few of us can afford this kind of expense, many become their own experts. If you decide to pursue this path, in my opinion, *food* as a source of nutrients is safe, and vitamin and mineral supplements are less so.

No vitamin ever came pure in nature. Vitamins are a single component in a complex of other vitamins and minerals. Look into any book on the composition of foods and see how many and varied are the vitamins and minerals (and maybe other nutrients we do not yet recognize) in a single food. Nuts and seeds are the closest we come to a hard, pellet form of food. These nuts and seeds are, again, a composite of nutrients. They are almost invariably chewed well before being swallowed. Pills are not.

A vitamin or mineral tablet or perle can get stuck in the throat or can lie against the lining of the esophagus, stomach, or small intestine, causing flushing (in the case of vitamin C) or irritation. Potassium salts in tablet form have actually burned holes in the lining of the gut, and there are some people whose digestion is so poor, they pass tablets through the digestive tract whole, seeing

them full-size in the stool the next day. These are just a few in-
stances. They do not happen to everyone.

Your system may need more of a particular vitamin or mineral
than you are getting in your food. To guarantee absorption, try to
take supplements that may be prescribed for you in fluid form
when you can. If you are going to try to take a supplement in
tablet or perle form, take it with a meal, not on an empty stomach.
Take it with solid food, not liquids. Better yet, look in the lists in
Chapter 17 for the foods highest in the needed nutrients and rede-
sign your diet so you need no added supplements.

Taking Stock

Look at yourself honestly. Are you doing as much for yourself as
you want? Take a look at your unclad body in a full-length mirror,
early morning before gravity takes its toll. Use a small hand mirror
to see yourself from the side and the back. What do you see? Be
honest with yourself.

Is your weight changing as you wish?
Are you getting tighter?
Is your belly sagging?
Does your bottom hang?
Can you see fat bumps and pads under your skin?
Are you flabby?
Swing your arms around — are your upper arms still loose?
Is there fat over your upper hip? (Remember that what looks
   like fat on the upper thigh can be sagging buttock
   muscles.)
Do you have fat folds from your underarms to your waistline
   in back?
How's your chin line?
Is your skin color improving?

Inspect yourself inch by inch. Are you satisfied with what you see?
Are you doing what you can to make it work? Is it time to make
more changes?

Look to Your Future

Healthy, tight-muscled, bright-eyed. If you're not like that right now, one year from now you might be. You have every reason to look forward to a terrific new life and lifestyle — if you're really consistent!

You have the information now to be the boss of your own body and to design yourself; and to get closer to having the kind of body you've always wanted (unless you wanted someone else's).

You may have to make very small steps forward, according to your condition, but make some small step to improve your health every single day. Just a single added step each day, and in thirty days you will have improved your life enormously. To stop doing something harmful can be considered doing something good. Two-way improvement.

No matter what condition you are in or what age you are, you can change for the better! It may be relative, but no matter where you are right now, better *is* better.

Set the Habits for Your Family

We are all creatures of habit. It is very easy to succumb to poor family habits of eating and moving. In fact, when seen clearly, a lot of what we like to call heredity (that means you can't help it, can't do anything about it, right?) is simply patterns of eating or moving built in to the family at large. Sometimes aunts, uncles, grandmothers, especially if they come from the same community, where their influence on each other is strong, will have common eating, buying, exercising, and learning habits.

The Italians out of habit use a lot of olive oil. The Japanese out of habit eat a lot of fish. The Bedouins out of habit use a lot of grains. The Armenians out of habit use a lot of nuts and seeds. All true, and all very good habits.

On the other hand, there is one ethnic group that out of habit has such a high-protein diet that the people all tend to be constipated and as a result suffer from anal fissures. There is another ethnic group that eats enough smoked foods to cause a high incidence of stomach cancer. And of course there is another ethnic group that out of habit consumes so much animal fat that there is a high incidence of heart and blood vessel disease and overweight.

"Habit" means it has been learned and practiced. There is nothing to stop you from changing your habits, or from changing, or at least influencing toward change, your family's habits.

You can make healthy food so delicious everyone will prefer it over other food. For instance, Chinese food tastes so good almost everyone will eat vegetables prepared in a large variety of oriental-style dishes.

You can "forget" to buy trashy family favorites and instead make available (overdo in the beginning, it makes a good impression) some *good* goody that you hope they will adopt. Try home-made popcorn (it smells so good) and real-fruit popsicles. The brownies designed by Adelle Davis are good for the children (too many calories for most adults). Also try dates stuffed with nuts, real homemade gelatin-like desserts (use Irish moss) made with fresh fruits.

Take a walk each day, taking a single child or other member of the family with you for a private time to talk. Private talking time is hard to come by in a family. There are always other people, television, radio, telephone. Escape from the interruptions and at the same time develop better family relations. No family? Try it at lunchtime with a friend or after work with a neighbor. Psychologists have known for a long time that the tougher issues that people generally have trouble discussing are more easily approached when the other person is not looking directly at you. And two of you get to exercise! Free exercise!

There are many other ways to subtly influence or change family habits. Make them up as you go along. Keep all changes positive. Don't demand! Don't force! You will defeat your own attempts.

Diet Design

Do you feel you are ready to design a diet for yourself? In the following chapters, you will find the Recommended Dietary Allowances and the foods highest in each nutrient. You can use the lists in several ways:

- You can try using one of the diet strategies from Part II, but substitute some of the foods from the lists for the foods you like least in the diet, or just for variety.

- You can try making up your own original diet with all your favorite foods from the lists.
- The foods in the lists are arranged to cover a few that are very high in each particular nutrient. One study years ago showed that animals fed the least caloric food with the highest amount of nutrients were the ones who lived the longest and suffered least disease. Not all the best foods for you are those lowest in calories. But by balancing your foods carefully you can lower your calories, or raise your calories, according to whether you want to gain or lose weight, while filling your particular nutritional needs.
- If you don't find many of your favorite foods on the lists, your eating habits can probably stand changing. Do it gradually. Choose one new food a day and make it something you think you'll really like.
- To build the best food strategy possible, whether you are trying to lose or gain weight or just become better nourished, use those foods most concentrated in nutrients, the ones that appear on many lists.

If you keep the calorie level of each meal around 200 to 300, you can then afford five or six meals a day and can still stay healthy while you lose weight. If you are trying to gain weight, have fewer meals in each of which you have at least 400 to 600 calories, still of the very best food. You want to gain muscle and other healthy tissues, not just fat. If you have not inherited a large, muscular frame, you will need regular exercise, maybe even weight training, to enlarge the muscle cells, to help your body turn some of these good foods into muscle.

If you have tried some of the diet ideas in this book and have been faithfully keeping your record cards, you should have much new information about yourself, your appetites, your likes and dislikes, when you get hungry, and your calorie needs. You have available to you charts to keep track of your weight, nutrient charts to help you balance your intake of nutrients to your specific needs, and many pages of excellent foods from which to choose.

Try foods one after the other and discard the ones that you decide are not for you, whether for right now or maybe even forever. Choose foods:

- that you love
- that you are capable of chewing
- that you are capable of digesting with no discomfort
- that keep you regular
- that meet your personal calorie needs
- that are low in animal fats
- to which you are not allergic
- with no salt added
- with no sugar added
- that are not refined
- that fit your way of life

Choose amounts of food that do not make you feel too full or too empty. Choose to eat as often or as seldom as makes you comfortable and healthy.

Take notes! This is a serious learning process. You will not remember it all unless you note down comments on all new information that you discover about yourself where food is concerned. Once you've learned your good new ways of eating, they will have become habit and will need little conscious attention. Right now, this information deserves your full attention. It will be a simple process for you to improve your nutrition, improve your weight, enjoy eating, and get and keep a feeling of good health and well-being.

Keep It in Balance

In designing your ultimate diet, make sure you are meeting all your Recommended Dietary Allowances by checking the food sources lists in Chapter 17. It takes a while to arrange the diet you like best so that it is exactly right for you. Don't do your diet designing too rigidly. By knowing which of your favorite foods are also good for you, you'll be able to make instant substitutions if you're in a restaurant, for instance, or find at home that you've run out of a particular food. Make the most of the fact that you now have knowledge and control by enjoying treats when you choose to.

Once you have designed your eating plan to your satisfaction, continue to fill out cards for at least one week out of every six for a year or so. For the next year fill out cards (for a week) every three to six months. Keep the cards whenever you see any signs of a lack of control, such as nagging illnesses or fluctuations in weight or unacceptable changes in appearance.

It is your body! Keep it under your control. Sure, you'll age. But with your ultimate diet, you will help yourself age as healthily and gracefully as possible.

Life Insurance

Years and years are wasted by us, in and out of hospitals, nursing homes, and homes for the aged, waiting in vain for someone to do for us what we should have been doing for ourselves right along.

You know yourself best! You know your weaknesses, your strengths, your heredity, your habits, your way of life, what foods you prefer. You do know, you just haven't put it all together. Now with all the information available, you will have all the clues you need by which to make yourself more capable of controlling your body.

You will know what foods you need, how much food you need, and how best to burn up the calories. You must make the time to plan and to carry out the changes you need in your habits. Nobody *has* time. *Take* the time from whatever you must; use time in front of the television or when reading or talking on the phone to exercise, and use it as a gift to yourself for your future.

Taking care of yourself is a serious investment. This is the only real chance you get at life insurance. Give it your best shot.

❧ 17 ❧

Nutrient Needs,
Nutrient Sources

Food is a popular topic in these times. There are almost as many diets proposed as there are types of nutrients and all of them are very specific, like instruction manuals for complicated machines. Once you raise your nutrition awareness, you don't need such detailed instructions. Most diets, such as those for losing weight, ultimately fail. They are too restricted for most of us who like freedom of choice. Once we have lost a certain amount of weight we abandon the diet with a feeling of relief. We are on parole! And sooner or later most of us are back to our old feeding habits like junkies, who, having kicked the habit in confinement, are exposed again to the old temptations when they are free. Diets of deprivation, while providing a temporary glow of virtue, are not useful for the majority of us. However, few people mind adding other foods to their diet to replace the usual foods, rather than just subtracting the offending foods. And that is one reason for writing this book, to help you become more knowledgeable about food so that you can devise your own diet — not a diet of deprivation but a true food strategy that can become a comfortable, natural, and ongoing part of your life.

As has been emphasized throughout the pages of this book, the first priority of any eating strategy should be good nutrition. Once your nutritional needs are met, you can factor in other goals, such as weight loss, weight maintenance, or weight gain. You may in fact be totally satisfied with your weight or general appearance (though I doubt it) — in that case, you will find that good nutrition is its own reward, and you will have the satisfaction that comes from knowing that you are doing what you can to take good care of your body.

The pages that follow summarize the best current views on our needs for known food elements and offer lists of foods that are excellent sources of these nutrients. Get to know these foods and make them a regular part of your life.

The Recommended Dietary Allowances

Because the book *Recommended Dietary Allowances* is a key resource to persons who are interested in human nutrition, it is important that you understand what its recommendations really mean to you as an individual. *Recommended Dietary Allowances* is researched, written, and published for the benefit of the American public. You may want to own a copy; it is available from the National Academy of Sciences (see Bibliography). The following extracts should help you evaluate the nutrient levels referred to throughout this book and shown in the table on page 291.

What the RDA represent:

"The RDA are recommendations [established for healthy populations] for the average daily amounts of nutrients that *population groups* should consume over a period of time. RDA should not be confused with requirements for a specific individual. Differences in nutrient requirements of individuals are ordinarily unknown. . . . Nutritional requirements differ among individuals and from time to time for a given individual. They differ with age, sex, body size, and physiological state. Some are further influenced by level of activity and by the environment in which an individual lives. . . .

"For certain nutrients, the requirements may be assessed as the amount that will just prevent failure of a specific function or the development of specific deficiency signs — an amount that may differ greatly from that required to maintain maximum body stores. Thus there are differences of opinion about the criteria that should be used to establish requirements."

Meeting the RDA:

"RDA are presented as *daily* allowances in order to simplify dietary calculations. [But,] in estimating dietary adequacy, it would seem entirely acceptable to average intakes over a 5–8 day period. However, if nutrient intake is insufficient to meet requirements for a prolonged period, the ability to respond to trauma and illness may ultimately be lessened, and depletion and deterioration may eventually occur — despite the effectiveness of the various mechanisms that prolong survival."

Some special considerations:

"Special needs for nutrients arising from such problems as premature birth, inherited metabolic disorders, infections, chronic diseases, and the use of medications require special dietary and therapeutic measures. These conditions are not covered by the RDA. . . .

"The period of recuperation following illness, trauma, burns, and surgical procedures, during which body stores are being replenished and tissues restored, is probably comparable to a period of growth [when a higher intake of many nutrients is generally needed]."

On calorie intake:

"Recommended allowances for energy are estimates of the average needs of population groups, not recommended intakes for individuals. These needs vary from person to person and are not easily predictable without detailed information about physical characteristics and activity of the individual."

On calorie intake and nutritional needs in aging:

"Body composition changes throughout life, with fat increasing and metabolically active tissues being slowly reduced. . . . As a result, less food is needed to meet energy

Recommended Daily Dietary Allowances *

Designed for the maintenance of good nutrition of practically all healthy people in the U.S.A.

	Age (years)	Weight (lb.)	Height (in.)	Protein (gm)	Fat-Soluble Vitamins			Water-Soluble Vitamins							Minerals					
					Vita-min A† (IU)	Vita-min D (IU)	Vita-min E (IU)	Vita-min C (mg)	Thia-min (mg)	Ribo-flavin (mg)	Niacin (mg NE)†	Vita-min B-6 (mg)	Fola-cin‡ (mcg)	Vitamin B-12 (mcg)	Cal-cium (mg)	Phos-phorus (mg)	Mag-nesium (mg)	Iron (mg)	Zinc (mg)	Iodine (mcg)
Males	15–18	145	69	56	5000	400	14.9	60	1.4	1.7	18	2.0	400	3.0	1200	1200	400	18	15	150
	19–22	154	70	56	5000	300	14.9	60	1.5	1.7	19	2.0	400	3.0	800	800	350	10	15	150
	23–50	154	70	56	5000	200	14.9	60	1.4	1.6	18	2.2	400	3.0	800	800	350	10	15	150
	51+	154	70	56	5000	200	14.9	60	1.2	1.4	16	2.2	400	3.0	800	800	350	10	15	150
Females	15–18	120	64	46	4000	400	11.9	60	1.1	1.3	14	2.0	400	3.0	1200	1200	300	18	15	150
	19–22	120	64	44	4000	300	11.9	60	1.1	1.3	14	2.0	400	3.0	800	800	300	18	15	150
	23–50	120	64	44	4000	200	11.9	60	1.0	1.2	13	2.0	400	3.0	800	800	300	18	15	150
	51+	120	64	44	4000	200	11.9	60	1.0	1.2	13	2.0	400	3.0	800	800	300	10	15	150
Pregnant				+30	+1000	+200	+3	+20	+0.4	+0.3	+2	+0.6	+400	+1.0	+400	+400	+150	**	+5	+25
Lactating				+20	+2000	+200	+3	+40	+0.5	+0.5	+5	+0.5	+100	+1.0	+400	+400	+150	**	+10	+30

* Adapted from Committee on Dietary Allowances, Food and Nutrition Board, *Recommended Dietary Allowances* (ninth revised edition), Washington, D.C., 1980. The allowances are intended to provide for individual variations among most normal persons as they live in the United States under usual environmental stresses. Diets should be based on a variety of common foods in order to provide other nutrients for which human requirements have been less well defined.

† Vitamin A allowances are sometimes also given as retinol equivalents (RE). For adult men the RDA is 1000 RE, or 100 mcg retinol. For adult women the RDA is 800 RE, or 800 mcg retinol (pregnant and lactating women should add 200 mcg and 400 mcg, respectively).

‡ 1 NE (niacin equivalent) is equal to 1 mg of niacin or 60 mg of dietary tryptophan.

§ The folacin allowances refer to dietary sources as determined by *Lactobacillus casei* assay after treatment with enzymes (conjugases) to make polyglutamyl forms of the vitamin available to the test organism.

** The increased requirement during pregnancy cannot be met by the iron content of habitual American diets nor by the existing iron stores of many women; therefore the use of 30–60 mg of supplemental iron is recommended. Iron needs during lactation are not substantially different from those of nonpregnant women, but continued supplementation of the mother for 2–3 months after parturition is advisable in order to replenish stores depleted by pregnancy.

gm = gram   IU = international unit
mcg = microgram   mg = milligram

requirements, and, unless food choices are made with great care, the amounts of essential nutrients consumed are likely to be less than during the more active years and may fall below desirable levels."

On using food to get your nutrients:

"RDA are intended to be met by a diet of a wide variety of foods rather than by supplementation [vitamin and mineral tablets] or by extensive fortification of [adding vitamins and minerals to] single foods.

"Most, but not all, nutrients are tolerated well in amounts that exceed the allowances by as much as two or three times, and a substantial proportion of the population commonly consumes an excess over the RDA for several nutrients without evidence of adverse effects. However ... high intakes of a number of nutrients — such as vitamins A and D and certain trace elements — can be toxic.... [These excesses most often occur through taking vitamin or mineral supplements.] The Committee on Dietary Allowances is not aware of convincing evidence of unique nutritional benefits accruing from the consumption of a large excess of any one nutrient or combination of nutrients."

On interpreting the data:

"With limited information about requirements, about the variability of requirements [according to your digestion, your differences from another, your differences under different conditions, all the variables] and factors that may influence digestibility [how it was prepared, stored, packaged], allowances for many nutrients cannot be estimated directly from the available scientific knowledge, [and] judgment must be invoked in interpreting and extrapolating from the available information."

Another group of nutrients also dealt with in *Recommended Dietary Allowances* are some about which there is less information on which to base allowances. These nutrients are treated in terms of Estimated Safe and Adequate Dietary Intakes (ESAD) and recommendations are given in the form of ranges.

Estimated Safe and Adequate Dietary Intakes (ESAD)

Nutrient	ESAD for Adults
Biotin	100–200 micrograms
Chloride	1700–5100 milligrams
Chromium*	50–200 micrograms
Copper*	2–3 milligrams
Fluoride*	1.5–4 milligrams
Vitamin K	70–140 micrograms
Manganese*	2.5–5 milligrams
Molybdenum*	150–500 micrograms
Pantothenic acid	4–7 milligrams
Potassium	1875–5625 milligrams
Selenium*	50–200 micrograms
Sodium	1100–3300 milligrams

Source: Adapted from Committee on Dietary Allowances, Food and Nutrition Board, *Recommended Dietary Allowances* (ninth revised edition), Washington, D.C., 1980.
  * Since toxic levels may be only several times usual intakes, the upper levels for these nutrients as indicated here should not be habitually exceeded.

The diet strategies presented in Part II of this book revolve around the RDA nutrients and some ESAD nutrients and also take into account a number of other dietary recommendations, such as those concerning the proportion of carbohydrates, fats, and sugar in the diet. Most of these recommendations are based on the Dietary Goals for the United States, developed by the Senate Select Committee on Nutrition and Human Needs in 1977. The nutrient analysis that accompanies each diet plan shows clearly how the diet relates to these various recommendations.

Food Sources of Major Nutrients

The following pages provide lists of foods that are excellent sources of each of the nutrients for which there are established RDA or ESAD levels. Several other important dietary constituents, such as cholesterol, fiber, and unsaturated fatty acids, are also included. For quick reference the recommended level of intake of each is shown, generally the RDA for adults aged 23 to 50 (other age groups or pregnant or lactating women should check the RDA table) or the ESAD, for all adults. It is hoped that these lists will help you make wise choices in custom-designing your eating plan.

Be aware that some of the listed nutrients — sodium, fat, and cholesterol, for example — are regularly consumed *in excess* by most people, and in these cases the purpose of the food lists is to help you avoid overconsumption of problem nutrients.

A similar listing of several lesser-known nutrients, for which there is not enough information on which to base official recommendations, follows the major nutrients.

Nutrient Deficiencies

Each nutrient is accompanied by a list of symptoms often associated with a chronic deficiency in that nutrient. Few people in the United States are obviously deficient in nutrients, but there are many who are subtly lacking them. Correcting for individual deficiencies with foods high in those nutrients is easy and safe using the food lists. If you eat a varied diet, it is difficult to get too much of a particular nutrient when you're dealing with food sources, not so true with supplements. (Of course, in the case of such things as sodium, fats, and refined carbohydrates, we all see people overindulge every day.)

Please don't use the deficiency symptoms as an excuse to go overboard with self-diagnosis. Since any given symptom may arise from a number of causes (many unrelated to nutritional deficiency), you should consult a doctor or nutritionist if your symptoms don't respond to food or if you intend to make more than a few simple changes in your diet.

If you wish to adjust your diet to add more of a particular nutrient, I suggest you choose from the five or six items at the top of the food lists. The lists are arranged in order from most to least, so that the foods highest in the nutrient are at the top. However, if the foods near the top don't appeal to you, choose your favorite foods from the lists.

I have tried to arrange these lists for ease of use. Thus, they contain a dozen or so foods that are very high in each nutrient. Of course, there are other foods with lesser amounts. You can find them in the books mentioned in the Bibliography.

Measurement of Nutrients

None of the nutrient amounts in any food composition listing is exact. Amounts of nutrients differ from carrot to carrot, from fish to fish, from liver to liver, according to growing, shipping, storing, and preparation procedures. As the laboratories themselves tell us, they are doing their best, but the numbers can give *approximations* only. Trying to eat by the numbers is not only ungratifying but also unnatural. Get a rough idea of what works for you, play with it till you get it right, and then enjoy.

Think about home preparation. It's a free-for-all. Some will round a cup. Some will heap it. Some will level it. Some will use a measuring cup. Some will use a tea cup. Some will even use their hands to measure. Who is right? Everybody — as long as you're healthy. Few of us in our own kitchens measure exactly. It's okay to measure roughly. Just make sure to get a little more rather than a little less of high-nutrient, low-calorie foods.

A cup or two of raw spinach will be somewhere between one-quarter and three-quarters of a cup when cooked, according to whether you cook it a lot or a little, remove the stems or leave them on, chop the spinach, purée the spinach, or leave it whole. Is it important? Not as long as you never get too little of the needed nutrients in the right amounts for you. Most foods shrink in cooking. It is for that reason that you will find different amounts of nutrients and calories in raw and cooked foods in any food lists.

As food wilts or is heated, it generally loses some of its fluids and "body" and takes up less space. The number of calories in a cup or two of cooked greens is probably the same as the number in a quart bowl full of the same greens raw in salad. This is why many of us serve both cooked greens and salads at the same meals. The two together add more colors, textures, flavors, and nutrients.

Amounts measured are seldom the same twice even if the same person is doing the measuring. Measuring spinach from the same bag on the second day (because it's a little more wilted), you will be able to get more spinach in the cup. It will take more young, delicate, small leaves of spinach to fill a cup than it would if you used old, overgrown spinach. Again, we want to have a feel for rough estimates. There is no need for and no sense in rigidity in your attitudes toward food. So relax and have fun.

ABOUT NUTRIENT MEASUREMENTS

The numbers in the tables and food lists are usually rounded off. That means 35.4 becomes 35 and 35.6 becomes 36; or 1.54 becomes 1.5 while 1.56 becomes 1.6.

1000 micrograms	= 1 milligram
1000 milligrams	= 1 gram
100 grams	= ¼ pound (approximately)
100 grams	= 3½ ounces
4 ounces	= ¼ pound
8 ounces	= ½ pound

Food Sources of Major Nutrients

VITAMIN A
RDA (adults, aged 23–50): Women, 4000 IU   Men, 5000 IU

Selected Foods Highest in Vitamin A

Food	Amount	Vitamin A (IU)	Calories
lamb liver *	¼ lb.	57,268	154
beef liver *	¼ lb.	49,784	159
veal liver *	¼ lb.	25,515	159
carrot juice	1 cup	24,750	96
pumpkin	1 cup	15,860	81
sweet potato	1	9,230	161
turnip greens, cooked	1 cup	9,140	29
kale, cooked	1 cup	9,130	43
mango	1	8,060	135
dandelion greens, raw	½ lb.	6,350	142
papaya	1	6,122	117
beet greens, cooked	1 cup	6,100	24
carrots, cooked	1 cup	4,650	47
spinach	1 cup	4,460	14
pepper, sweet red, raw, sliced	1 cup	4,450	31

* When adding these very high animal sources of vitamin A to your diet, remember that once a week is generally plenty.

Deficiency Symptoms

foamy patches on white of eye
night blindness
drying and coloration of
   conjunctiva
dry mouth, lack of saliva
dry patches on mucous
   membrane
rough dry skin
scaly skin
lined skin
elephant skin (elbow, knee, and
   instep)

bumpy skin (toad skin)
opaque corneas
coloring in whites of eyes
thickening of conjunctiva
skin blemishes
sties on edge of eyelid
diarrhea
loss of appetite
dry nose
sinus headache
atrophic vaginitis (dry vagina)
some gastrointestinal disorders

VITAMIN B-1 (Thiamin)
RDA (adults, aged 23–50): Women, 1.0 mg   Men, 1.4 mg

Selected Foods Highest in Vitamin B-1

Food	Amount	Vitamin B-1 (mg)	Calories
peas, raw	1 cup	0.51	122
wheat germ, raw	¼ cup	0.5	91
rice, polish, bran	¼ cup	0.5	70
collards, raw, with stems	½ lb.	0.46	91
peas, cooked	1 cup	0.45	114
dandelion greens, raw	½ lb.	0.43	102
kale, with stems	½ lb.	0.37	120
beef heart, braised	¼ lb.	0.3	213
asparagus, cut, raw	1 cup	0.24	35
lobster, cooked	½ lb.	0.23	216
turnip greens, cooked	1 cup	0.22	29
okra, raw	1 cup	0.17	36

Deficiency Symptoms

fatigue	retarded growth
apathy	numbness in legs
loss of appetite	electrocardiogram abnormalities
nausea	inflammation of nerves
moodiness	emaciation
irritability	edema
depression	changed heart function

VITAMIN B-2 (Riboflavin)
RDA (adults, aged 23–50): Women, 1.2 mg   Men, 1.6 mg

Selected Foods Highest in Vitamin B-2

Food	Amount	Vitamin B-2 (mg)	Calories
veal liver	¼ lb.	5	296
beef kidney, braised	¼ lb.	5	286
beef liver, cooked	¼ lb.	5	260
chicken liver, cooked	1 cup	2.4	219
beef heart, braised	¼ lb.	1	213
collards, raw, with stems	½ lb.	0.7	45
mushrooms, canned, drained	1 cup	0.66	51
kale, raw, with stems	½ lb.	0.55	120
mustard greens, raw	½ lb.	0.5	70
broccoli, raw	½ lb.	0.5	72
turnip greens, cooked	1 cup	0.35	29
mushrooms, raw, diced	1 cup	0.32	20
broccoli, cooked	1 cup	0.31	40
asparagus, cut, raw	1 cup	0.27	35
spinach, cooked, drained	1 cup	0.25	41

Deficiency Symptoms

fissures at corners of mouth and
   eyes (sore, split skin)
whistle marks
swollen, puffed lips
shiny red tongue

fissures of tongue
yellow, fatty plugs in pores
   around nose
crusty, oily, scaly skin
beriberi

VITAMIN B-3 (Niacin)
RDA (adults, aged 23–50): Women, 13 mg   Men, 18 mg

Selected Foods Highest in Vitamin B-3

Food	Amount	Vitamin B-3 (mg)	Calories
tuna, water-packed	½ lb.	30	288
chicken breast	1 avg.	29	250
swordfish, broiled	½ lb.	23	371
shad, American, cooked	½ lb.	20	456
tuna in oil, drained	1 cup	19	315
trout, rainbow	½ lb.	19	442
veal liver	¼ lb.	19	296
halibut, broiled	½ lb.	18	388
mackerel	½ lb.	18	433
beef heart, braised	¼ lb.	8	213
rice, polish, bran	¼ cup	7.5	70
turkey, light meat, cooked	¼ lb.	7	213
chicken livers, cooked	1 cup	6.2	219
mushrooms, canned, drained	1 cup	5.4	51
mushrooms, raw, diced	1 cup	5.4	51
kale, raw, with stems	½ lb.	5	120
chicken thigh	1 avg.	5.1	199
collards, raw, with stem	½ lb.	4	90
wheat bran, raw	¼ cup	3	50
broccoli, raw	½ lb.	2.05	73
asparagus, cut, raw	1 cup	2	35

Deficiency Symptoms

yellow, fatty plugs in pores around nose
eczema
inflamed tongue
skin looks sunburned
skin discoloration
swollen, puffed lips
pellagra
dermatitis of areas exposed to sunlight
inflammation of mucous membranes
diarrhea
rectal irritation
irritability
anxiety
depression
hallucination
confusion
disorientation
stupor

VITAMIN B-6 (Pyridoxine)

RDA (adults, aged 23–50): Women, 2.0 mg   Men, 2.2 mg

Selected Foods Highest in Vitamin B-6

Food	Amount	Vitamin B-6 (mg)	Calories
chicken breast	¼ lb.	1.2	96 (est.)
beef liver, cooked	¼ lb.	0.95	260
chicken liver, cooked	1 cup	0.82	219
banana, raw	1 avg.	0.66	105
kale, raw, with stems	½ lb.	0.65	120
chicken back	1 avg.	0.6	96 (est.)
carrot juice	1 cup	0.5	96
Brussels sprouts, raw	½ lb.	0.5	102
broccoli, raw	½ lb.	0.43	72
tomato juice	1 cup	0.37	46
spinach, cooked, drained	1 cup	0.34	41
pepper, sweet green, raw, sliced	1 cup	0.21	18
asparagus, cut, raw	1 cup	0.2	35
chicken drumstick	1 avg.	0.2	104 (est.)
squash, summer, raw	1 cup	0.19	25
cauliflower, raw, sliced	1 cup	0.17	23
chicken wing, roasted	1 avg.	0.15	50 (est.)
spinach, raw	1 cup	0.14	14
watercress, raw, chopped	1 cup	0.14	24

Deficiency Symptoms

inflammation of lining of eye
fissures at corner of mouth
tongue inflamed and shiny
fissures of tongue
eczema
bumpy skin (toad skin)

yellow, fatty plugs in pores
  around nose
greasy, scaly skin
muscle weakness
irritability
depression

VITAMIN B-12 (Cobalamin)
RDA (adults, aged 23–50): 3 mcg

Selected Foods Highest in Vitamin B-12

Food	Amount	Vitamin B-12 (mcg)	Calories
beef liver, cooked	¼ lb.	91	260
beef kidney, braised	¼ lb.	70	286
veal liver	¼ lb.	68	296
oysters	6 oz.	30	114
chicken liver, cooked	1 cup	27	219
liverwurst	1 oz.	24	93
crab, steamed	½ lb.	23	211
mackerel	½ lb.	20	433
beef heart, braised	¼ lb.	13	213
chicken heart, cooked	1 cup	11	268
trout, rainbow	½ lb.	12	443
herring (8 per lb.)	1 lrg.	5	99
oysters	1 oz.	5	19
tuna, water-packed	½ lb.	5	288
beef tongue	¼ lb.	4	277
veal sweetbreads	1 oz.	4	48
sardines, oil-packed	1 oz.	3	58
sand dab	½ lb.	3	179
scallops, steamed	½ lb.	3	254
haddock	½ lb.	3	179

Deficiency Symptoms

aching feet

burning feet

throbbing feet

tender calves

inflammation of tongue and mouth

degeneration of nervous system

neuritis

sore tongue

loss of weight

back pains

apathy

mental and nervous abnormalities

neck and arm pain

sciatic pain

BIOTIN
ESAD (all adults): 100–200 mcg

Selected Foods Highest in Biotin

Food	Amount	Biotin (mcg)	Calories
chicken livers, simmered	100 grams	170	165
beef liver	(about	96	222
calves' liver, fried	3½ oz.)	53	261
peanut butter		39	585
walnuts, English or Persian, chopped		37	694
peanuts		34	585
chocolate, bitter		32	505
sardines, in brine or mustard, with liquid		24	186
eggs, fried		20	210
almonds, shelled		18	638
cauliflower, raw		17	27
mushrooms, raw		16	28
salmon, canned, with liquid		15	124
chicken, broiled		11	136
oysters, canned, with liquid		9	73
whole wheat flour, hard wheats		9	361
spinach, frozen, chopped, leaf		7	25
corn, raw, sweet white		6	96

Deficiency Symptoms

dry, scaly dermatitis	pale skin
loss of appetite	depression
nausea	decreased production of red blood cells
vomiting	
muscle pains	higher blood cholesterol levels
shiny red tongue	seborrheic dermatitis

VITAMIN C (Ascorbic Acid)
RDA (adults, aged 23–50): 60 mg

Selected Foods Highest in Vitamin C

Food	Amount	Vitamin C (mg)	Calories
acerola, raw	½ cup	822	15
kale, raw, with stems	½ lb.	422	120
broccoli, raw	½ lb.	257	73
Brussels sprouts, raw	½ lb.	232	102
mustard greens, raw	½ lb.	220	71
collards, raw, with stems	½ lb.	209	91
currants, black, raw	1 cup	203	71
pepper, hot green, chili	1 cup	167	49
guava, raw	1 avg.	165	45
pepper, sweet red, raw, sliced	1 cup	163	25
broccoli, cooked	1 cup	140	40
Brussels sprouts, cooked	1 cup	135	56
pepper, sweet green, sliced, cooked	1 cup	130	24
parsley, raw, chopped	1 cup	103	26
pepper, sweet green, raw, sliced	1 cup	102	18
turnip greens, cooked	1 cup	100	29
watercress, raw, chopped	1 cup	99	24
strawberries, raw	1 cup	84	45
cauliflower, raw, sliced	1 cup	66	23
pimientos, canned	2 oz.	54	15
cabbage, red, raw, sliced	1 cup	43	22

Deficiency Symptoms

bleeding gums	mild to severe hemorrhages
swollen gums	fatigue
easy bruising	weight loss
loosening teeth	irritability
losing teeth	shortness of breath
anemia	small hemorrhages under skin
spider veins	poor wound healing
weakness	malformed bones
pain in joints	fragility of capillaries
degeneration of muscle fibers	heart failure

CALCIUM
RDA (adults, aged 23–50): 800 mg

Selected Foods Highest in Calcium

Food	Amount	Calcium (mg)	Calories
wakame	3½ oz.	1300	265
kale, with stems	½ lb.	565	120
collards, raw, with stems	½ lb.	461	91
dandelion greens, raw	½ lb.	424	102
mustard greens, raw	½ lb.	415	71
yogurt, lowfat, plain	1 cup	415	144
cheese, Parmesan, grated	1 oz.	398	129
milk, skim	1 cup	302	86
turnip greens, cooked	1 cup	267	29
broccoli, raw	½ lb.	234	73
watercress, raw, chopped	1 cup	189	24
broccoli, cooked	1 cup	136	40
parsley, raw, chopped	1 cup	122	26
endive, raw	1 cup	41	10

Deficiency Symptoms

menstrual cramps
air swallowing
indigestion
insomnia
inability to relax
irritability of muscles
hampered ability of muscles to
  contract
hypersensitivity to pain
tendency to hemorrhage (need
  calcium for blood to clot)
cataracts
tooth decay

complications in childbirth
inability to regulate nutrients
  and other ions in and out of
  cell membranes
fracturing of bones
weak, brittle bones
osteoporosis
stunting of growth
malformation of bones
rickets
osteomalacia
tetany
kidney stones

CHLORIDE
ESAD (all adults): 1700–5100 mg

Selected Foods Highest in Chloride

seaweeds	scallops
clams	table salt
oysters	

Deficiency Symptoms

slow, shallow breathing	lack of appetite
listlessness	convulsions (occasional)
muscle cramps	

CHOLESTEROL
Recommended Intake: 300 mg daily, maximum

If you have a blood cholesterol problem, a level which is 190 milligrams or more, you may want to keep away from the following list of foods. An elevated blood cholesterol level should be met with a vegetarian diet, devoid of all but nonfat dairy products, eggs, and even all shellfish, at least till control is regained. Since your body manufactures all the cholesterol it needs, cholesterol deficiency is not a problem—cholesterol excess *is*.

Selected Foods Highest in Cholesterol

Food	Amount	Cholesterol (mg)	Calories
chicken livers, cooked	1 cup	883	219
lobster, cooked	½ lb.	491	216
chicken heart, cooked	1 cup	350	268
shrimp, raw	½ lb.	340	208
chicken gizzard, cooked	1 cup	281	222
egg, raw, boiled, poached	1 lrg.	274	79
egg yolk	1 lrg.	272	63
crab, steamed	½ lb.	227	211
chicken back, raw	1 avg.	210	96 (est.)
clams, canned, drained	1 cup	128	157
cod-liver oil	1 TBSP.	119	126
veal sweetbreads	1 oz.	123	48
caviar, sturgeon	1 oz.	63	74
beef kidney, braised	¼ lb.	86	286
veal liver, raw	¼ lb.	50	296

CHROMIUM
ESAD (all adults): 50–200 mcg

Selected Foods Highest in Chromium

Food	Amount	Chromium (mcg)	Calories
blackstrap molasses	100 grams	115	213
eggs	(about	52	163
cheese, hard	3½ oz.)	51	370
liver		50	140
wheat bran		40	213
beef, lean, raw		32	180
wheat, whole grain		29	330
wheat germ		25	363
potatoes, raw		24	76
oysters, Eastern, raw		20	66
chicken		14	107
cornmeal, dry		11	364
banana		11	85
spinach, raw		9	26
carrots, raw		8	42
orange		5	50
beans, green		4	32
strawberries		3	37
mushrooms, raw		3	28
milk, skim		1	36

Deficiency Symptoms

impaired glucose tolerance
reduced effectiveness of insulin
atherosclerosis
cataracts
growth retardation
heart disease
high blood fats

impotence
frigidity
low resistance to infections
neurological disorders
high blood sugar levels
adult onset diabetes

COPPER
ESAD (all adults): 2–3 mg

Selected Foods Highest in Copper

Food	Amount	Copper (mg)	Calories
oysters, raw	100 grams	13.7	66
calves' liver, fried	(about	12	261
lamb liver, broiled	3½ oz.)	10	261
blackstrap molasses		6	213
pork liver, fried		2.5	241
Brazil nuts		2.4	654
lobster		1.8	95
sunflower seeds		1.8	560
walnuts, English		1.4	651
almonds		1.4	598
wheat germ, toasted		1.3	391
wheat bran		1.3	213
pecans		1.1	687
wheat germ		0.7	363
lamb leg, roasted, broiled		0.7	266
peanut butter		0.6	582
apricots, dried		0.5	260
beans, red, raw		0.5	343
turnip greens, raw		0.4	30
avocado, raw		0.4	167
collards, raw, with stems		0.3	40
beef, lean, raw		0.2	180

Deficiency Symptoms

anemia
skeletal defects
demyelination and degeneration
  of nervous system
defects in pigmentation and
  structure of hair

reproductive failure
pronounced cardiovascular
  lesions
elevated serum cholesterol

VITAMIN D
RDA (adults, aged 23–50): 200 IU

Selected Foods Highest in Vitamin D

Food	Amount	Vitamin D (IU)	Calories
herring, Atlantic, raw	100 grams	900	176
sardines, canned, drained	(about	752	187
salmon, red, canned	3½ oz.)	420	114
tuna, oil-packed, drained		232	197
all livers		14–67	165–261
all other fatty fish		varies	varies

Deficiency Symptoms

rickets
decalcification of bones
tetany
osteomalacia
enlarged joints
bowed legs
knock-knee

beadlike projections on each side
  of chest
bulging forehead
potbelly
delayed eruption of temporary
  teeth

VITAMIN E
RDA (adults, aged 23–50): Women, 11.9 IU   Men, 14.9 IU

Selected Foods Highest in Vitamin E

Food	Amount	Vitamin E (IU)	Calories
kale, raw, with stems	½ lb.	18	120
corn oil	1 TBSP	11	120
cucumber	1 cup	8	16
wheat germ, raw	¼ cup	7	91
hazelnuts (filberts), shelled	¼ cup	7	214
almonds, shelled	10 avg.	6	212
safflower oil	1 TBSP	5	120
sesame oil	1 TBSP	4	120
asparagus, cut, raw	1 cup	3	35
turnip greens	1 cup	3	29
chard, raw	½ lb.	3	57
mango	1 avg.	3	135
peas	1 cup	3	122
chocolate, bitter	1 oz.	3	143
Brussels sprouts, raw	½ lb.	3	102

Deficiency Symptoms

stiff joints
intermittent claudication
increased red blood cell fragility
decreased endurance
edema
skin lesions

blood abnormalities
inability to absorb fat
shortened red blood cell life span
increased urinary excretion of
    creatinine

FIBER

Recommended Intake: 6 gm crude fiber or more daily (actual needs vary widely)

Most food composition tables still show crude fiber content of foods, so this is the measure used in this book. Crude fiber is only one component of *dietary* fiber, which is more difficult to measure. Speaking very roughly, the total dietary fiber content of grains is about three times the crude fiber figure; fruits and vegetables contain about 50 percent more total fiber than the crude fiber figure indicates. The National Cancer Institute recommends consuming 25 grams of dietary fiber daily.

Selected Foods Highest in Fiber

Food	Amount	Crude (gm)	Calories
oat bran	1 oz.	8	110
artichoke, globe, boiled	1 avg.	7	35
blackberries, raw	1 cup	6	74
raspberries, red, raw	1 cup	4	61
dandelion greens, raw	½ lb.	4	102
Brussels sprouts, raw	½ lb.	4	102
broccoli, raw	½ lb.	3	73
pumpkin, canned	1 cup	3	81
Brussels sprouts, cooked	1 cup	2	56
broccoli, cooked	1 cup	2	40
cucumber, raw	1 lrg.	2	45
beans, green, cooked	1 cup	1	31
pepper, sweet green, raw, sliced	1 cup	1	18
cauliflower, raw, sliced	1 cup	1	23
wheat bran	1 TBSP	1	32

Deficiency Symptoms

constipation
diverticulosis
tears in lining of bowel

anal fissures
bloating

FLUORIDE
ESAD (all adults): 1.5–4 mg

Selected Foods Highest in Fluoride

dried seaweed	smoked herring
tea	wheat germ
mackerel	crab
shrimp	
sardines	
salmon	

Deficiency Symptoms
excess dental caries
maybe increased osteoporosis

FOLACIN (Folic Acid)
RDA (adults, aged 23–50): 400 mcg

Selected Foods Highest in Folacin

Food	Amount	Folacin (mcg)	Calories
bulgur, dry	1 cup	7926	628
chicken liver, cooked	1 cup	1077	219
beef liver, cooked	¼ lb.	249	260
collards, raw, with stems	½ lb.	232	91
Brussels sprouts, raw	½ lb.	177	102
spinach, cooked, drained	1 cup	164	41
broccoli, raw	½ lb.	157	73
beets, diced, cooked	1 cup	153	54
kale, raw, with stems	½ lb.	136	120
beets, diced, raw	1 cup	126	58
spinach, raw, chopped	1 cup	110	14
lettuce, looseleaf	1 cup	95	10
broccoli, cooked	1 cup	87	40
parsley, chopped, raw	1 cup	70	26
cabbage, Chinese, raw	1 cup	62	11
watercress, raw, chopped	1 cup	61	24
beans, green, raw	1 cup	53	35

Deficiency Symptoms

megaloblastic anemia
  (of infancy)
macrocytic anemia
  (of pregnancy)
lowered white blood cell count

sore, red, smooth tongue
diarrhea
poor growth
mental deterioration
burning, painful feet

IODINE
RDA (adults, aged 23–50): 150 mcg

It is worth noting that you do not want either too much or too little
iodine. A high intake of dairy products can give you too much iodine.

Selected Foods Highest in Iodine

Food	Amount	Iodine (mcg)	Calories
kelp, dried	3½ oz.	62,400	230
salt, iodized		7600	0
fish, saltwater		330	103
vegetables (est.)		30	20–50
milk and milk products (est.)		14	50–66
eggs		13	157
whole-grain wheat, oats		9	360

Deficiency Symptoms
goiter

coarse hair

high blood cholesterol

obesity

dry skin

IRON
RDA (adults, aged 23–50): Women, 18 mg   Men, 10 mg

Selected Foods Highest in Iron

Food	Amount	Iron (mg)	Calories
veal liver	¼ lb.	16	296
oysters, canned	1 cup	13	158
chard, raw	½ lb.	7	56
mustard greens, raw	½ lb.	7	70
dandelion greens, raw	½ lb.	7	102
oysters, fresh	3 oz.	6	58
parsley, raw, chopped	1 cup	4	26
spinach, cooked, drained	1 cup	4	41
beet greens, cooked, drained	1 cup	3	26
cucumber, raw	1 lrg.	3	45
spinach, raw, chopped	1 cup	2	14
watercress, raw, chopped	1 cup	2	24
beans, green, cooked	1 cup	2	32
beans, yellow, cooked	1 cup	2	32
wheat bran, raw	¼ cup	2	50

Deficiency Symptoms

rapid heartbeat
pale gums
pale mucous membrane
shortness of breath
easy tiring
lightheadedness
insomnia
headache
pale skin

blurred vision
fissures at corner of mouth
tongue inflamed and shiny
concave nails
anemia
fatigue
sensitivity to the cold
tingling fingers and toes

VITAMIN K
ESAD (all adults): 70–140 mcg

A healthy body synthesizes its own vitamin K from intestinal bacteria.

Selected Foods Highest in Vitamin K

Food	Amount	Vitamin K (mcg)	Calories
turnip greens	100 grams	650	28
broccoli	(about 3	200	26
lettuce	3½ oz.)	129	15
cabbage		125	24
beef liver		92	222
spinach		89	26
asparagus		57	20
watercress		57	19
pork liver		25	241
oats		20	390
peas, green		19	71
wheat, whole grain		17	357
beans, green		14	24
pork tenderloin		11	254
eggs		11	157
peaches, raw		8	38
ground beef		7	301
chicken liver		7	165

Deficiency Symptoms
delayed blood clotting

MAGNESIUM
RDA (adults, aged 23–50): Women, 300 mg   Men, 350 mg

Selected Foods Highest in Magnesium

Food	Amount	Magnesium (mg)	Calories
snails	3½ oz.	250	90
chard, raw	½ lb.	147	56
spinach, canned, drained	1 cup	129	49
collards, raw, with stems	½ lb.	129	90
soy flour, low fat	½ cup	127	156
tofu (soybean curd)	3½ oz.	111	72
wheat germ, raw	¼ cup	84	91
kale, raw, with stems	½ lb.	83	120
dandelion greens, raw	½ lb.	81	102
wheat bran, raw	¼ cup	70	50
mustard greens, raw	½ lb.	61	70
spinach, raw, chopped	1 cup	48	14
okra, raw	1 cup	41	36
watercress, raw, chopped	1 cup	25	24
squash, summer, raw	1 cup	21	25
cauliflower, raw, sliced	1 cup	20	23
beans, green, cooked, drained	1 cup	18	32

Deficiency Symptoms

depression
irritability
nervousness
convulsions
muscle spasms
smooth muscle spasms (lump in throat)
convulsions
tetany
kidney stones
calcium deposits in organs and soft tissues
vertigo
heart abnormalities
alcoholic hallucination during withdrawal
swollen gums
decreased potassium levels
decreased calcium levels
anorexia
nausea
vomiting
inability to synthesize lecithin
atherosclerosis
inhibited utilization of fats and cholesterol
menstrual cramps
hysteria (anxiety attacks)
hyperventilation

MANGANESE
ESAD (all adults): 2.5–5 mg

Selected Foods Highest in Manganese

Food	Amount	Manganese (mg)	Calories
rice bran	100 grams	34.7	276
rice polish	(about	17.1	265
walnuts, English	3½ oz.)	15.2	651
wheat germ		13.3	363
wheat bran		11	213
rice, whole grain		9.6	360
molasses, blackstrap		4.3	213
wheat, whole grain		3.7	330
oats, whole grain		3.7	390
soybeans, dry		3	403
peanuts, roasted		2.5	582
sunflower seeds		2.3	560
beans, navy, dry		2.1	340
barley, whole grain		1.2	349
lettuce		1	18
potatoes, raw		1	76

Deficiency Symptoms

decreased production of various
   enzymes
retarded growth
hyperactivity
abnormal bone structure
joint deformities
poor equilibrium

uncoordinated movements
male impotence
female sterility
aggravation of growth
   impairments
abnormal metabolism of lipids

MOLYBDENUM
ESAD (all adults): 150–500 mcg

Selected Foods Highest in Molybdenum

Food	Amount	Molybdenum (mcg)	Calories
lima beans, dry	100 grams	323	345
wheat germ	(about	210	391
liver	3½ oz.)	150	165–220
green beans		67	25
whole wheat flour		48	361
poultry		40	170 (est.)
spinach		25	25
cabbage		17	20

Deficiency Symptoms
unknown

PANTOTHENIC ACID
ESAD (all adults): 4–7 mg

Selected Foods Highest in Pantothenic Acid

Food	Amount	Pantothenic Acid (mg)	Calories
calves' liver, fried	100 grams	8	261
beef liver, fried	(about	7.7	222
beef heart, lean, braised	3½ oz.)	2.5	179
peanut butter		2.5	585
peanuts		2.4	581
mushrooms, raw		2.2	28
salmon, steamed		1.8	197
egg, hard-boiled		1.7	157
pecans		1.7	739
rice, brown, cooked		1.5	119
lobster, boiled		1.5	119
sunflower seeds		1.4	560
cashews		1.3	596
broccoli		1.1	26
chicken, stewed		1.2	183
peppers, sweet		1.1	18
avocados		1.1	67

Deficiency Symptoms

irritability
restlessness
loss of appetite
indigestion
abdominal pains
nausea
headache
sullenness
depression
fatigue
weakness

numbness
tingling of hands and feet
burning sensation in feet
insomnia
respiratory infections
rapid pulse
staggering gait
increased reaction to stress
increased sensitivity to insulin
decreased gastric secretions
decreased antibody production

PHOSPHORUS
RDA (adults, aged 23–50): 800 mg

Selected Foods Highest in Phosphorus

Food	Amount	Phosphorus (mg)	Calories
flounder (sole), cooked	½ lb.	780	458
scallops, steamed	½ lb.	766	254
cod, broiled	½ lb.	621	385
smelt, raw	½ lb.	617	222
haddock	½ lb.	447	179
sand dabs	½ lb.	442	179
wheat germ, toasted	¼ cup	323	108
rice, polish or bran	¼ cup	290	69
wheat germ, raw	¼ cup	279	91
milk, skim	1 cup	247	86
mushrooms, canned, drained	1 cup	243	51
wheat bran, raw	¼ cup	182	50
broccoli, raw	½ lb.	177	72
sardines, canned in oil	1 oz.	141	58
mushrooms, raw, diced	1 cup	81	20
watercress, raw, chopped	1 cup	68	24

Deficiency Symptoms

loss of appetite
anorexia
stiff joints
fragile, easily broken bones
loss of energy, weakness
malaise

bone pain
demineralization of bone
muscular weakness
rickets
osteomalacia

POTASSIUM
ESAD (all adults): 1875–5625 mg

Up to three times the ESAD amount may be ingested regularly without trouble unless you have kidney problems.

Selected Foods Highest in Potassium

Food	Amount	Potassium (mg)	Calories
chard, raw	½ lb.	1248	57
bamboo shoots, raw	½ lb.	1209	61
broccoli, raw	½ lb.	867	73
mustard greens, raw	½ lb.	855	72
spinach, cooked, drained	1 cup	583	41
tomato juice	1 cup	552	46
beet greens, cooked, drained	1 cup	481	26
cucumber, raw, whole	1 lrg.	481	45
parsley, raw, chopped	1 cup	436	26
asparagus, cut, raw	1 cup	375	35
watercress, raw, chopped	1 cup	353	24
apricots, raw	3 avg.	313	51
tomato, raw	1 avg.	300	27
mushrooms, raw, diced	1 cup	290	20
radishes, red, raw	10 avg.	261	14
spinach, raw, chopped	1 cup	259	14
cauliflower, raw, sliced	1 cup	251	23
cabbage, Chinese, raw	1 cup	190	11
endive, raw	1 cup	147	10
lettuce, looseleaf	1 cup	145	10

Deficiency Symptoms

muscle weakness
flabbiness
fatigue
poor intestinal tone, bloating
  and constipation
heart abnormalities
weakness of respiratory muscles
impaired glucose and protein
  metabolism
fluid retention
high blood pressure

low blood sugar
ringing in ears (tinnitus)
vertigo
headache
abnormal electrocardiogram
irritability
possible paralysis
nausea
vomiting
diarrhea
swollen abdomen

PROTEIN
RDA (adults, aged 23–50): Women, 44 gm   Men, 56 gm

Selected Foods Highest in Total Protein

Food	Amount	Protein (gm)	Calories
tuna, water-packed	½ lb.	64	288
shrimp, canned, drained		55	263
halibut		48	227
bluefish		47	266
pollock		46	216
snapper		45	211
sea bass		44	211
abalone		43	223
haddock		42	179
smelts		42	223
shrimp, fresh		41	207
catfish		40	234
cod		40	177
crab, meat only		39	211
flounder, sole		38	179
lobster, fresh meat		38	207
sand dabs		38	179
chicken breast		37	197
turkey, young		36	240
scallops, steamed		35	184

Deficiency Symptoms

hair changes color
hair can be painlessly plucked
enlarged liver
muscles small and flabby
darkening and flaking of skin
underweight
edema (fluid retention)
anemia

diarrhea
apathy
weakness
gut disturbances
susceptibility to disease
"tomcat" look—swelling jawline
 at sides of face

SELENIUM
ESAD (all adults): 50–200 mcg

Selected Foods Highest in Selenium

Food	Amount	Selenium (mcg)	Calories
smelts, raw	100 grams	123	98
wheat germ	(about 3½ oz.)	111	363
lobster		104	95
Brazil nuts		103	654
pork kidneys		64	106
wheat, whole grain		63	330
wheat bran		63	213
clams		55	82
crab		51	93
oysters, raw		49	66
pork		42	243
rye, whole grain		37	334
lamb		30	201
turnips, raw		27	30
swiss chard, raw		26	25
blackstrap molasses		26	213
garlic		25	137
oats, whole grain		21	390
barley, whole grain		18	349

Deficiency Symptoms

cancer
heart disease
damaged blood vessels
cataracts
premature disintegration of red
  blood cell membranes
increased susceptibility to
  infections
fluid accumulation in male testis
feeble and broken sperm cells
liver disease
pancreatic disease

SODIUM
ESAD (all adults): 1100–3300 mg

Sodium deficiencies are uncommon. Watch out for excess!

Selected Foods Highest in Sodium *

Food	Amount	Sodium (mg)	Calories
kombu (seaweed)	3½ oz.	2500	219
cottage cheese, dry	1 cup	918	123
rice, brown, cooked, salted	1 cup	767	178
cheddar cheese	1 oz.	701	112
lobster	½ lb.	680	207
scallops	½ lb.	578	184
roquefort cheese	1 oz.	513	111
corn grits, cooked, salted	1 cup	502	125

* See page 257 for a more extensive listing of foods high in sodium.

Deficiency Symptoms

reduction of plasma volumes
lassitude
weakness
muscle cramps
vomiting

elevated blood urea
reduced growth
loss of appetite
weight loss
headache

UNSATURATED FATTY ACIDS

Recommended Intake: About 20% of total daily calories (on a 2000-calorie diet, this translates to about 44 gm a day); of this, a maximum of 10% daily calories should be polyunsaturated fatty acids, with 1–2% of calories as linoleic acid

All foods that contain unsaturated fatty acids easily become rancid when the food is chopped and left to stand (as in chopped nuts), when it is roasted (as in roasted nuts and seeds), or when these oils are removed from their original packaging, such as pressed nut and seed oil. It is best to use the whole fresh food or to buy small, sealed bottles of fresh oils and keep them tightly covered and refrigerated between uses. Always smell bottles of oil before use. The slightest smell of rancidity should be cause for them to be thrown away. Rancid oils are destructive to your body.

Selected Foods Highest in Polyunsaturated Fatty Acids (PUFA)

Food	Amount	PUFA (gm)	Calories
walnuts, English	100 gm	42	651
Brazil nuts	100 gm	25	654
pignolias	100 gm	23	552
eel	½ lb.	15	528
peanuts, roasted	100 gm	14	582
mackerel	½ lb.	13	433
peanut butter	100 gm	12	582
salmon	½ lb.	11	492
safflower oil	1 TBSP	10	124
almonds	100 gm	10	598
sunflower oil	1 TBSP	8.9	124
soybean oil	1 TBSP	8.1	124
herring	½ lb.	8	399
whitefish	½ lb.	8	351
corn oil	1 TBSP	7.8	124
cottonseed oil	1 TBSP	7.1	124
wheat germ	100 gm	7	363

Selected Foods Highest in Linoleic Acid

Food	Amount	Linoleic Acid (gm)	Calories
walnuts, black	100 gm	37	628
walnuts, English	100 gm	35	651
sunflower seeds	100 gm	30	560
Brazil nuts	100 gm	25	654
pignolias	100 gm	22	552
pumpkin seeds	100 gm	20	553
squash seeds	100 gm	20	553
Spanish peanuts	100 gm	16	585
peanut butter	100 gm	15	582
almonds	100 gm	10	598
safflower oil	1 TBSP	10	124
corn oil	1 TBSP	7	124
cottonseed oil	1 TBSP	7	124
soybean oil	1 TBSP	7	124
sesame oil	1 TBSP	6	124

Deficiency Symptoms

decreased production of sex and adrenal hormones

decrease of valuable intestinal bacteria

imperfections in every cell structure

dry, lifeless hair

scaly, rough skin

ZINC
RDA (adults, aged 23–50): 15 mg

Selected Foods Highest in Zinc

Food	Amount	Zinc (mg)	Calories
oysters, fresh, raw	1 oz.	20	19
lobster, cooked	½ lb.	18	216
oat flakes, dry	3½ oz.	14	387
pine nuts	3½ oz.	14	636
crab, steamed	½ lb.	10	211
veal liver	¼ lb.	7	296
chicken liver, cooked	1 cup	6	219
chicken gizzard, cooked	1 cup	6	222
beef liver, cooked	¼ lb.	6	260
lean beef loin	3½ oz.	5.7	164
whole wheat flour	3½ oz.	5.5	331
wheat germ, toasted	¼ cup	5	108
wheat germ, raw	¼ cup	3	91
spinach, canned, drained	1 cup	2	49
chicken drumstick	1 avg.	2	193
sprouts, mung, raw	1 cup	2	37
asparagus, cut, raw	1 cup	1	35
spinach, cooked, drained	1 cup	1	41
sprouts, alfalfa, raw	1 cup	1	41
mushrooms, raw, diced	1 cup	1	20

Deficiency Symptoms

loss of appetite
stunted growth
skin changes
small sex glands
loss of taste
lightened pigment of hair

dull hair
white spots on fingernails
delayed healing of wounds
malformed offspring
enlarged prostate

Food Sources of Other Nutrients

Listed below are several nutrients for which research has not yet established a dietary need in humans. This does not mean that a need may not exist, only that the need has not been established.

CHOLINE

The Committee on Dietary Allowances does not recommend at this time any human allowance of choline. In general, we get 500–900 mg per day in our average diets.

Selected Foods Highest in Choline

Food	Amount	Choline (mg)	Calories
eggs	100 grams	527	157
liver, all varieties	(about	356	136
wheat germ	3½ oz.)	306	391
soybeans		290	405
cabbage, raw		254	24
wheat bran		188	353
navy beans		168	340
rice polish		122	265
rice bran		122	276
oats		101	283
wheat, whole grain		101	360
hominy		99	358
rice, whole grain		93	363
turnip greens		91	30
barley, whole grain		90	305
blackstrap molasses		74	230
corn, whole grain		54	348

Deficiency Symptoms

Some nutrition experts claim these as choline deficiency symptoms in mammals, although they have not been reported in humans.

enlarged liver
fatty liver

hemorrhagic kidney damage
poor growth

INOSITOL

As with choline, experts disagree as to our needs for inositol. We seem to be capable of synthesizing what we need. Average daily intake is about 300–1000 mg.

Selected Foods Highest in Inositol

Rich Sources	Good Sources
citrus fruits	bran
blackstrap molasses	fruits
heart	legumes
kidney	milk
liver	muscle meats
wheat germ	nuts
	vegetables
	whole grains

Deficiency Symptoms

retarded growth	loss of hair

VITAMIN P (Bioflavonoids)
There are no recommendations for bioflavonoids at this time.

Since most research shows that vitamin C and bioflavonoids work best together, the idea of getting your daily intake from foods is logical. Many nutrition experts agree that bioflavonoids have a helpful effect different from that of vitamin C.

Selected Foods Highest in Vitamin P
The following foods are generally recognized as being the richest sources. They are not necessarily in order. On all citrus fruits, bioflavonoids are highest in the white parts inside the rind and the center core of white.

apricots	grapefruit	peppers
blackberries	grapes	plums
black currants	lemons	rose hips
broccoli	oranges	tangerines
cantaloupe	papaya	tomatoes
cherries		

Deficiency Symptoms

tendency to bleed (hemorrhage)	increased arthritic response
capillaries break easily	increased inflammation
easy bruising	
hemorrhaging around hair follicles	

PARA-AMINOBENZOIC ACID (PABA)
Our need for para-aminobenzoic acid has not been established.

Selected Foods Highest in Para-Aminobenzoic Acid (PABA)
These foods are generally recognized as the richest sources.

eggs	peanuts
fish	soybeans
liver	wheat germ
molasses	

Deficiency Symptoms

nervousness	headache
fatigue	constipation
irritability	digestive disorders
depression	

SULFUR

There are no Recommended Dietary Allowances for sulfur, as the requirement is related to and involved with the amino acids, the structural units of protein. Requirement is met when the intake of amino acids methionine, cysteine, and cystine is adequate.

Selected Foods Highest in Sulfur

Food	Amount	Sulfur (mg)	Calories
peanuts	100 grams	380	582
blackstrap molasses	(about	350	230
pork chops, lean	3½ oz.)	300	254
Brazil nuts		290	715
turkey		290	190
sardines, in oil, drained		310	246
beef, lean		270	220
lamb, shoulder roast, lean		240	205
wheat germ		240	391
navy beans, dry		230	340
soybeans, dry		220	405
wheat bran		220	353
salmon, canned		220	124
oats, whole grain		210	283
beans, lima, dry		200	359
rice bran		180	276
rice polish		170	265
wheat, whole grain		160	360
barley		150	305
almonds		150	598

Deficiency Symptoms

retarded growth

Postscript

Miraculous as our bodies are in self-repair, the system does not work well without the needed raw materials, the nutrients. We need not only the energy that food provides but also many factors that our bodies can't manufacture for themselves. Many of these factors are not ordinarily abundant even if we were to live directly off the land. For example, there is little or no iodine in East German or Swiss soil, no calcium in crops raised on some volcanic islands, no sodium in the interior of any large body of land except in small pockets. Furthermore, among animals we humans are genetically unique in that we don't make our own vitamin C but have to get it from what we eat.

Agriculture and transportation make possible an adequate diet for all of us who live in Western countries. There need be no deficiencies, yet they are still common. Our caloric needs have changed in recent generations because manual labor has been replaced by powered machinery, walking has been replaced by riding, and we are shielded from the elements by heated houses. We need in general only half or two-thirds the calories per day as was needed only a hundred years ago. Those of us who still eat in the old-fashioned manner tend to get fat on the excess calories. Those of us who eat only what we need in calories tend to get less of the other nutrients that are also an essential part of food.

The situation is further complicated by the fact that food-processing for distribution and storage almost always removes many nutrients while preserving calories and "acceptable appearance."

With all these influences on our diet we can still eat better and preserve our health better than our ancestors if we know how to pick and choose among the wealth of food available to us. There is no reason of age, illness, or accident to prevent us from eating what we need not only to stay alive but to preserve our bodies in best nutritional condition. We can lose or gain weight, recover from illness or accident, or avoid foods to which we are sensitive and yet get all the nutrients that are necessary for the body to function best. All that we require is the information, so that we may select foods not only by nutritional composition but also according to our tastes.

That is what this book is about. For in the end it is you — not your doctor, family, or teacher — who is responsible for your health. And when illness or accident or age hits you, how you are affected depends very much on how you attend, with changes in nutrition and in movement, to your body.

Bibliography

The lists of foods and nutrients throughout this book were compiled from a number of sources, cited below. Because the sources were of varying usefulness in drawing up any given list in this book, you may find what appear to be inconsistent data in some of the listings. This is unavoidable, since nutrient values can vary considerably from source to source, depending on how calculations were done and on the specific food samples tested. As mentioned elsewhere in this book, all such values can at best be approximations, and for the purposes of drawing up a well-balanced diet program these approximations are entirely adequate. Persons wishing more detailed information about nutrient values should go directly to these sources:

Church, C. F., and Church, H. N. *Food Values of Portions Commonly Used.* 12th ed. Philadelphia: J. B. Lippincott, 1975.

Ensminger, A. H., et al. *Foods and Nutrition Encyclopedia.* 2 vols. Clovis, California: Pegus Press, 1983.

Etheridge, R. Health-Aide (nutrition software). San Rafael, California: Programming Technology Corporation, 1982.

Kirschmann, J. D., and Dunne, L. J. *Nutrition Almanac.* 2nd ed. New York: McGraw-Hill, 1984.

Leveille, G. A., Zabik, M. E., and Morgan, K. J. *Nutrients in Foods.* Cambridge, Massachusetts: The Nutrition Guild, 1983.

Rao, M. N., and Polacchi, W. *Food Composition Table for Use in East Asia.* Part II, *Amino Acid, Fatty Acid, Certain B-Vitamin, and Trace Mineral Content of Some Asian Foods*. Food Policy and Nutrition Division, Food and Agriculture Organization of the United Nations, unpublished (c. 1975).

Watt, B. K., and Merrill, A. L. *Composition of Foods: Raw, Processed, Prepared*. Agriculture Handbook No. 8. Washington, D.C.: U.S. Department of Agriculture, 1963. (Available from Superintendent of Documents, U.S. Government Printing Office, Washington, D.C. 20402.)

The following works were also consulted in the preparation of this book:

Committee on Dietary Allowances, Food and Nutrition Board, National Research Council. *Recommended Dietary Allowances*. 9th ed. Washington, D.C.: National Academy of Sciences, 1980. (Available from Office of Publications, National Academy of Sciences, 2101 Constitution Avenue N.W., Washington, D.C. 20418.)

Gilman, A., et al., eds. *The Pharmacological Basis of Therapeutics*. 6th ed. New York: Macmillan, 1980.

Goodhart, R. S., and Shils, M. E. *Modern Nutrition in Health and Disease*. 6th ed. Philadelphia: Lea & Febiger, 1980.

Lentner, C., ed. *Geigy Scientific Tables*. 8th ed. Vol. 1. West Caldwell, New Jersey: Ciba-Geigy Corp., 1981.

McArdle, W. D., Katch, F. I., and Katch, V. L. *Exercise Physiology*. 2nd ed. Philadelphia: Lea & Febiger, 1986.

Index

Acidophilus, 47, 219. *See also* Milk products
Activity, *see* Physical activity
Addiction, carbohydrate, 53–54. *See also* Carbohydrates; Cravings and binges
Additives, 18–19, 20–21, 28, 259, 264, 265, 268–69
  MSG, 45, 254
  preservatives, 18, 158, 250, 255, 266
  See also Processed food; Salt; Sugar
Advertising, 6, 19
Aerobics, *see* Physical activity
Agene, 21. *See also* Additives
Aging
  as "disease," 123
  and nutrient loss, 5, 34, 38, 128, 259, 290–92
  and osteoporosis, 126
  and physical activity, 5, 206, 208
  and special diets, 23, 35, 125, 127, 182, 234, 287
Alcohol, *see* Beverages
Allergies, 28, 42, 43, 45–48, 90, 242
  and fluid retention, 211
  and substitution in diet of another food, 105, 220, 234, 238, 239
Aluminum cans, 170. *See also* Processed food
Aluminum pots and pans, 233. *See also* Cooking methods and equipment
American Heart Association, 106
Amino acids, *see* Protein

Amylase, 180. *See also* Saliva
Anal spasms, 70, 85
Animal fat, *see* Fats
Anorexics, 196
Antibiotics, *see* Medication
Anti-Stress Diet, *see* Shine (Anti-Stress) Diet
Apathy: as diet side effect, 139
Appetite vs. hunger, 10–11
Arctic Circle, 35, 36
Arthritis, 123. *See also* Illness
Ascorbic acid, *see* Vitamin C
Auden, W. H., 69

Backache, 126–27. *See also* Illness
Barley: allergy to, 47. *See also* Allergies
Basic Grain Cereal (recipe), 240
Basic High-Potassium Soup, *see* High-Potassium Soup, Basic
Behavior disorders: DES and, 20
"Belly bloppers" (exercise), 87–88. *See also* Physical activity
Beverages, 248–49
  alcoholic, 27, 54, 260
  juices, *see* Fruits, canned or bottled; Fruits, fresh; Vegetables, fresh
  soft drinks
  See also Milk products; Soups and broths; Two-Minute Diet; Water
Binges, *see* Cravings and binges
Bioflavonoids, *see* Vitamin P
Biotin: sources and deficiency symptoms (table), 303

Blackstrap molasses, 88
Blender/juicer/processor, use of
    for cereal, 241
    and roughage, 90, 175, 182
    for soup, 174, 175, 182, 229, 235
    in Two-Minute Diet, 128, 135
    and vegetable juice, 227, 230, 235,
        249, 251, 281
Blood pressure, *see* High blood pressure
Body type, 4–6, 198
Bone loss, *see* Osteoporosis
Bone Stock, 235, 249
    importance of, 228, 231
    recipe, 232–33
Bowel movements, *see* Constipation;
    Diarrhea
Bran, *see* Fiber (roughage)
Breads, 219, 256, 260, 261
    nutrient analysis (table), 238–39
    See also Flour; Grains
Buckwheat: allergy to, 47. *See also* Al-
    lergies
Butter, buttermilk, *see* Milk products
"Butter yellow," 20

Cabbage family, *see* Vegetables, fresh
Calcium
    absorption, citric acid and, 28
    deficiency, 38, 125–27, 139, 140,
        304, 335
    -magnesium balance, 47, 138
    sources (milk and nonmilk products),
        28, 47, 88, 105, 140, 173, 231–
        34 *passim*, 261, (table) 305
    storage and loss, 24, 26, 45, 104, 126–
        27, 138, 253
    tranquilizing effect, 28
    See also Minerals
Calories
    burned by diet change, 40
    burned by physical activity, 22, 193–
        97, 200–201, 206, 214, 237–38,
        (table) 198–99
    and calorie-counting as false basis for
        diet planning, 7
    carbohydrates and, 53, 236–38
    cholesterol intake based on, 107
    daily needs, 7–8, 22, 50, 51, 66, 126,
        212, 285, 290, 335
    in eight basic (core) diets, 51, 66, 82,
        101, 120, 135, 153, 169, 179
    fat/calorie content of selected foods
        (tables), 237, 242–44, 262–64,
        267, 275–78

    in High-Nutrient Soup, 66
    intake vs. output (sample record
        card), 191, 217
    and low-calorie diet, *see* Lean, Clean
        Machine Diet
    and low- or no-calorie salad dressings,
        see Salads and dressings
    vs. nutrients ("X-" vs. "A-"rated), 22–
        23, 36, 51, 217–20, 235–49, 285
    in processed food, *see* Processed food
    recommended intake (table), 50
    recording intake/output of, 190–94,
        197–99, 201, 216–19, 249
    in restaurant foods, 13, 218
    size and frequency of meals and, 25,
        26, 285
    sources (tables), 236–44, 262–64,
        267, 275–78
        fats and oils, 39, 141, 193–94, 261–
            66
        meats, 242–43, 260, 266, 267
Cancer, 20–21. *See also* Illness
Canned food, *see* Fruits, canned or bot-
    tled; Processed food; Vegetables,
    canned
Can openers, "throwaway," 170. *See
    also* Cooking methods and equip-
    ment
Carbohydrates, 120
    addiction to, 53–54
    in "A-rated" foods (tables), 236–40
    complex, 69, 237–40
    high-carbohydrate vegetables (table),
        238
    indigestible, 69 *(see also* Fiber [rough-
        age])
    low-carbohydrate diets, *see* High-
        Protein, Low-Carbohydrate Diet;
        Lean, Clean Machine Diet
    minimum requirements, 53
    no- and low-carbohydrate foods
        (nutrient analysis tables), 242–44
    refined, 23, 27, 44, 53, 54, 250, 259,
        294
    saliva and, 280
    unrefined, 27, 34, 53–54
Carcinogens, 20–21
Cards, *see* Record-keeping
Carrot juice, 251, 281. *See also* Vegeta-
    bles, fresh
Cellulose, 69. *See also* Fiber (roughage)
Cereal
    and constipation, 86, 88
    recipes for, 240–42

Checklists, charts, *see* Record-keeping
Cheese, 38
  tranquilizers in combination with, 21
  See also Milk products
Chicken, *see* Poultry
Chloride: sources and deficiency symp-
    toms (table), 306
Chocolate: additives to, 21. *See also* Ad-
    ditives
Choice Filler Foods, 51–52, 225–35
Cholesterol
  in anti-stress diet, 35, 106–7, 120
  in high-protein diet, 139–40
  recommended intake, 106–7, 307
  sources (and reduction of), 35, 106–
    7, 219, 264, 293
    dairy products, 28, 47
    fish or chicken vs. meat or eggs, 36,
      39, 107, 140, 242, 263
    foods highest in (table), 307
Choline: sources and deficiency symp-
    toms (table), 330
Chromium: sources and deficiency
    symptoms (table), 308. *See also*
    Minerals
Circulatory ailments, 211. *See also* High
    blood pressure
Citric acid: and calcium, 28
Cobalamin, *see* Vitamin B-12
Cobalt, 22. *See also* Minerals
Cod-liver oil, 106, 140. *See also* Oils
Colon, 85–86, 88, 90
Condiments: sugar in, 260
Constipation, 17, 34–35, 69–70, 85–
    88, 139, 140. *See also* Regularity
    Diet
Cooking methods and equipment
  aluminum pots and pans, 233
  can openers, 170
  and cooking water, *see* Water
  deep-frying, 38
  double boiler, 71
  and measurements, 295–96
  pressure cooker, 71, 230, 231, 232,
    233, 250–51
  and removal of fat, 38, 219, 232, 234,
    242
  roasting of nuts and seeds, 237, 241,
    327
  steaming, 219, 226, 250
  stir-frying, 219, 227
  See also Blender/juicer/processor, use
    of
Copper: sources and deficiency symp-

toms (table), 308. *See also* Min-
    erals
Corn products, 87, 237, 260–61
  allergy to, 47
  See also Grains
Coronary artery disease, 39. *See also* Ill-
    ness
Cosmetics: chemical agents in, 21
Cramps, *see* Muscle Spasms
Cravings and binges, 27, 274
  and carbohydrate addiction, 53–
    54
Cysteine, 334
Cystic mastitis, 28
Cystine, 334

Dairy products, *see* Milk products
Davis, Adelle, 284
Deep-frying, 38. *See also* Cooking meth-
    ods and equipment
Deficiency or depletion of soil, 21–22,
    253, 335
Deficiency symptoms, 259, 297–334.
    See also Digestive problems; Ill-
    ness
Dehydration, 211–12
DES (diethylstilbestrol), 20
Desserts, 14–15, 247–48, 284
DHA (docosahexaenoic acid), 140
Diabetes, 123, 139, 208, 259. *See also*
    Illness
Diarrhea, 45, 70, 90. *See also* Digestive
    problems
Diet(s)
  aging and, *see* Aging
  basic assumptions about food used in,
    38
  change in, and weight loss, 40–41
  checklist for, *see* Record-keeping
  choice of, 6–9, 24, 34–43, 188–89,
    201–2, 203–4, 282–87, 336
  cost of, 41, 269
  "customizing," 16–17, 27–29, 33–
    34, 49–52, 189, 284–87, 288 (*see
    also individual diets*)
  "excuses" against, 9, 12
  exercise combined with, *see* Physical
    activity
  habits and, *see* Habits
  high-fat, 35
  and illness, *see* Illness
  liquid, *see* Two-Minute Diet
  reasons for, 33–36
  right, importance of, 7–8

Diet(s) *(cont.)*
 side effects (possible, of high-protein
   diet), 139
 unsuitable for women, *see* Women
 See also High-Protein, Low Carbohydrate Diet; Lean, Clean Machine
   Diet; Pocket Diet; Raw Diet; Regularity Diet; Shine (Anti-Stress)
   Diet; Sweet Diet; Two-Minute
   Diet; Vegetarian diet; Weight loss
Dietary Allowances, Committee on,
   292. *See also* Recommended Dietary Allowances (RDA)
Dietary Goals for the United States, 293
Dietary supplements, *xv–xvi*, 41, 44,
   174, 281–82, 293
 toxicity of, 28, 292
 See also Minerals; Vitamins
digestive problems
 aging and, 127–28, 259
 allergies and, 45 *(see also* Allergies)
 and raw food or roughage, 35, 87, 90,
   174–75, 182, 235
 See also Constipation; Diarrhea; Illness; Saliva; Teeth and gums
Disease, *see* Illness
Double boiler, 71. *See also* Cooking
   methods and equipment
Dyes, toxic, 19, 21, 28. *See also*
   Toxicity

Ectomorph (body type), 4
Eggs: cholesterol content of, 107, 219
Electrolytes, 139, 225. *See also* Calcium;
   Magnesium; Potassium
Endomorph (body type), 4
Environmental pollution, *see* Pollution
Enzymes, 45
 salivary, 89, 280
EPA (eicosapentaenoic acid), 140
Epilepsy, 21, 28. *See also* Illness
Estimated Safe and Adequate Dietary In-
   takes (ESAD), 23, 292–93, 303,
   306, 308–9, 313–26 *passim*
"Excuses," *see* Diet(s)
Exercise, *see* Physical activity

Fast food, 157
Fasting, 40, 126, 138–39
Fat/calorie content of selected foods, *see*
   Calories
Fatigue: as diet side effect, 139
Fats
 animal, 39, 107, 140, 216, 219

 as calorie source, 39, 141, 193–94,
   261–66 *(see also* Calories)
 and cholesterol, 39, 107, 140, 263
 and high-fat diet, 35
 overconsumption of, 39, 44, 261,
   265, 293, 294
 in processed foods, 158, 218, 252,
   262, 263, 266, 269
 rancidity of, 141 *(see also* Rancidity)
 removal of, in cooking, 38, 219, 232,
   234, 242
 saturated, and avoidance of, 36, 107,
   153–54, 261, 262
 stored, metabolism of, 244
 See also Oils
Fatty acids, polyunsaturated (PUFA),
   140, 237
 sources and deficiency symptoms
   (table), 327–28
Fat weight, *see* Weight
Fava beans, toxicity of, 19. *See also*
   Toxicity
Fiber (roughage), 45, 229, 268, 269
 digestive problems precluding, 35, 87,
   90, 174–75, 182, 235
 and peristalsis, 35, 69, 85–87, 139
 sources, 173, 227, 261
   bran, 17, 70, 86–87, 88
   cereals, 88, 240, 242
   vegetables, 69, 86, 230
 sources and deficiency symptoms
   (table), 312
Field, Dr. Richard T.: quoted, 16
Figs, 70. *See also* Fruits, dried
Fish and shellfish, 38
 allergy to, 45
 bone stock from, 231, 233
 as calorie source, 243, 263, 275, 276,
   277
 canned, 129, 160
 and cholesterol, 36, 39, 106, 107, 140,
   263
 fatty, 140, 154
 freshwater, 89, 242
 as oil source, 216, 265
 oysters as zinc source, 66, 173, 228,
   329
 raw, 89
"Flab," 196, 213. *See also* Muscles
Flavorings, *see* Additives; Herbs and
   spices; Salt; Sugar
Flour
 white, 17, 21, 27, 218, 260
 whole wheat, 260, 261

See also Breads; Grains
Fluid retention or loss, *see* Water
Fluoride: sources and deficiency symptoms (table), 313
Folacin (folic acid), 38, 135
  sources and deficiency symptoms (table), 314
Food
  "A-" vs. "X-rated," 217–20, 225, 235–49, 252
  as celebration or love offering, 7, 14–15
  "Choice Filler," 51–52, 225–35
  choice of, 285–86 *(see also* Diet[s])
  cravings for, *see* Cravings and binges
  diet, basic assumptions about, 38
  eating habits, *see* Habits
  enjoyment of, *xvii*, 6–7, 204–5, 279–80
  "fake," 264–69
  "fast" vs. "junk," 157
  natural, toxicity of, *xii*, 18–19, 249
  preparation of, *see* Cooking methods and equipment
  sensitivities to, *see* Allergies
  taste preferences and dislikes, 43, 46, 174, 209
  and temptations, 9, 10, 13, 42
  See also Processed food; Restaurant food; *individual foods*
Food dyes, 19, 20, 28
Food sources of major nutrients (tables), 293–334
Fried foods, *see* Cooking methods and equipment
Fructose (fruit sugar), 54. *See also* Sugar
Fruits, canned or bottled, 129, 160, 219, 260, 269
  as calorie source, 277
  juices, 55, 129, 160, 219, 258
Fruits, dried, 54, 70, 241, 260
Fruits, fresh, 13, 38, 219, 250, 264
  as calorie source, 54, 236, 243, 275–78
  and constipation, 69, 86, 87, 88
  cooked vs. raw, 86, 90
  in desserts, 248
  juices, 209, 260, 281
  as mineral source, 86, 140
  nutrient analysis (table), 236

Garnishes, 231, 235
Gelatin salads, dressings, and desserts,

230, 245, 248. *See also* Salads and dressings
Glycogen, 39–40
Gout, 139. *See also* Illness
Grain, Nut, and Seed Cereal (recipe), 241
Grains, 264
  allergies to, 47–48, 220, 238, 239
  as calorie source, 276, 278
  and cholesterol, 264
  grain cereal recipes, 240–42
  refined, 17, 252, 260–61, 268
  wheat germ, 17, 101, 174, 228
  whole, 38, 86–87, 216, 219, 250, 265, (nutrient analysis table) 239
  See also Corn products; rice products

Habits, 5, 8, 31, 127, 203
  of eating, 11, 53, 204–5, 209–10, 219, 225, 274, 283–84, 285, 288
  of movement, 205–6, 208–9, 284, 287
Hair dyes, 21
Hair loss, 138
Headaches, MSG allergy, 45. *See also* Allergies
Heart disease, 39, 139, 253, 264. *See also* Illness
Hemorrhoids, 87
Hepatitis: pollution and, 89
Herbs and spices
  with beverages/soups, 128, 175, 210, 229, 235, 274
  with legumes, 240
  in salads and dressings, 247
  as salt substitute, 254
  usefulness of, *xi–xii*, 250, 280
Herb teas, 249. *See also* Beverages
Heredity, 42, 188, 283
  and toxicity, 18–19
High blood pressure, 211
  constipation and, 87
  fat/calories and, 39
  salt and, 45, 253, 256, 258
  See also Illness
High-carbohydrate vegetables: nutrient analysis (table), 238. *See also* Carbohydrates; Vegetables, fresh
High-Nutrient Soup, 51, 105, 173, 174, 228
  calorie content of, 66
  as diet supplement (tables), 64–66, 80–81, 99–100, 118–19, 133–34, 151–52, 167–68, 177–78

High-Nutrient Soup (*cont.*)
  High-Potassium Soup based on, 176,
    227, 228
  nutrient analysis (tables), 64–65
  variations on, 229–31, 234–35
High-Potassium foods, 227, 249, 258
  nutrient analysis (table), 226
  See also Potassium
High-Potassium Soup, Basic, 244, 249
  additions to, 230
  as calcium source, 105
  High-Nutrient Soup based on, 176,
    227, 238
  nutrient analysis (table), 229
  preparation time, 41, 227
  recipe, 228
  as stress fighter, 106
  as vegetable source, 43
High-Protein, Low-Carbohydrate Diet,
    35–36, 51, 138–56, 228, 231
Holiday food, 14
Hormones
  animals treated with, 20
  hormonal balance (in women), 126
  hormonal differences between men
    and women, 138, 212
  hormonal reactions, 18, 20, 211,
    215
  as medication, 278
Hot baths, 211, 258
Hunger, 10–11, 52
Hypoglycemia (low blood sugar), 54
Hypothyroidism, 48

Illness
  allergy and, 48 (*see also* Allergies)
  diet and, 3–4, 35, 36, 39, 123–24,
    125, 139
  and frequency of meals, 24–25
  kidney problems, 21, 139, 211, 253,
    259
  progressive diseases, 123–24
  and RDA, 290
  See also Deficiency symptoms; Diges-
    tive problems; High blood pres-
    sure; Stress; Toxicity; *specific
    illnesses*
Inositol: sources and deficiency symp-
    toms (table), 331
Intrinsic factor, 259
Iodine, 335
  sources and deficiency symptoms
    (table), 315
Irish moss, 235, 245, 284

Iron
  deficiency/need in women, 38, 66,
    82, 101, 120, 135, 169, 179,
    291n
  depletion of, from soil, 21
  sources, 66, 82, 88, 101, 135
  sources and deficiency symptoms
    (table), 316

Juices, *see* Fruits, canned or bottled;
    Fruits, fresh; Vegetables, fresh
Junk food, 157

Kefir, 47. *See also* Milk products
Ketosis, 138–39
Kidneys, 254
  and kidney problems, 21, 139, 211,
    253, 259

Laban, 47. *See also* Milk products
Labeling, *see* Processed food
Lactation, *see* Women
Laxatives and suppositories, 85, 87–88.
    See also Constipation
Lean, Clean Machine Diet, 36, 40, 51,
    173–83, 227, 228
Legumes, 38, 250
  allergy to, 239
  and cholesterol, 264
  nutrient analysis (table), 240
Light: nutrients destroyed by, 159
Linoleic acid, 327
  sources and deficiency symptoms
    (table), 328
Liquid diet, *see* Two-Minute Diet
Liver, *see* Meats
Low blood sugar, 54
Low-calorie diet, *see* Lean, Clean Ma-
    chine Diet
Low-calorie foods (table), 275–78
Low-carbohydrate diets, *see* High-
    Protein, Low-Carbohydrate Diet;
    Lean, Clean Machine Diet
Low- or no-calorie salad dressings, des-
    serts, and beverages, 230, 245–51,
    265–66, 274
Low- or no-carbohydrate foods:
    nutrient analysis (table), 242–44
Lunch meats, *see* Meats

Magnesium, 279
  -calcium balance, 47, 138
  and constipation, 85, 86, 87, 88
  sources, 86, 88, 140, 173, 261

sources and deficiency symptoms
(table), 318
storage and loss, 38, 85, 104, 138,
139, 140, 253
tranquilizing effect, 28
Manganese: sources and deficiency
symptoms (table), 319. *See also*
Minerals
Margarine, 48, 141
Massachusetts Institute of Technology,
195
Mayonnaise, *see* Salads and dressings
Meals
enjoyment of, *see* Food
size and frequency of, 24–27, 204,
250, 279, 285
Measurements, 295–96. *See also* Cooking methods and equipment
Meats
and cholesterol, 106, 107
cured (sugar in), 260
fat/calorie content (tables), 262, 267
fish or chicken substituted for, 36, 39,
140, 154
hormone-treated, 20
lean, in diet, 38, 39, 242
liver, 107, 174, 228
lunch, 256, 262, 266, 267
See also Processed food
Medication, 211, 278, 290
antibiotics, 47, 69
See also Physician, consultation with
Men
calcium deficiency in, 126
calories needed or burned by, 51, 66,
125–26, 199
and cholesterol, 120
and High-Protein Diet, 35, 138
muscle weight in, 212
protein needs of, 81, 179
RDA for, 64–65, 291
vitamin and mineral needs of, 66, 82,
101, 153, 169, 179, 291n
and weight-loss programs, 278
Ménière's disease, 256. *See also* Illness
Menopause, 126, 258, 278
Menstruation, 126, 138, 207
premenstrual diet, 105
premenstrual weight gain, 278
Menus, 49
High-Protein, Low-Carbohydrate
Diet, 143–50
Lean, Clean Machine Diet, 176
Pocket Diet, 161–66

Raw Diet, 92–98
Regularity Diet, 71–79
Shine (Anti-Stress) Diet, 109–17
Sweet Diet, 56–63
Two-Minute Diet, 129–32
Mesomorph (body type), 4
Metabolism changes, 139, 194–95, 208,
219, 290–92
Methionine, 334
Michaelson, Charlotte, 245
Milk products
allergy to, 28, 45, 47, 105, 234
butter, buttermilk, 47, 48, 141
as calcium source, 28, 47, 105
as calorie source, 263, 276, 278
cheese, 21, 38
cultured products, 45, 47, 69, 219
and iodine, 315
pasteurized, 47
on shopping lists, 55, 70, 91, 108,
129, 160
skim, in diet, 38
yogurt, 47, 69
Minerals
diets supplying, 35, 140
RDA of, 64
removed in processing, 269
soil depletion or deficiency, 21–22,
335
sources, 86, 140, 231, 235, 281
sources and deficiency symptoms
(tables), 308, 309, 316–29 *passim*
storage and loss, 24, 126
supplementary, 44, 255, 281–82,
292
See also Calcium; Iron; Magnesium;
Potassium; Zinc
Mirrors, use of, 5–6, 282
Molasses (blackstrap), 88
Molybdenum: sources and deficiency
symptoms (table), 320. *See also*
Minerals
MSG (monosodium glutamate), 45, 254.
See also Additives
Multiple sclerosis, 123, 208. *See also* Illness
Muscles
diet and, 34, 196
exercise and, 195–96, 197, 204, 206,
212–14, 285
muscle tone, 5, 34, 197, 206, 213–15
muscle weight, 211, 212, 285
and "weight faker," 211
Muscle spasms, 70, 85, 105

Nasal stuffiness, 45. *See also* Allergies

National Academy of Sciences, 44, 289

National Cancer Institute, 312

Natural food, toxicity of, *xii*, 18–19, 249. *See also* Toxicity

Nausea: as diet side effect, 139

Niacin, *see* Vitamin B-3

Nightshade family, 238

No-calorie salad dressing, 247. *See also* Salads and dressings

No-carbohydrate foods: nutrient analysis (table), 242–43

Nutrient analysis, 49, (tables) 297–334

  breads, 238–39

  fresh fruits, 236

  high-carbohydrate vegetables, 237–38

  High-Nutrient Soup, 64–65

  High-Potassium Foods, 226

  High-Potassium Soup, 229

  High-Protein, Low-Carbohydrate Diet, 151–52

  Lean, Clean Machine Diet, 177–78

  legumes, 240

  low-carbohydrate foods, 243–44

  no-carbohydrate foods, 242–43

  nuts and seeds, 237, 241

  Pocket Diet, 167–68

  Raw Diet, 99–100

  Regularity Diet, 80–81

  Shine (Anti-Stress) Diet, 118–19

  Sweet Diet, 64–65

  Two-Minute Diet, 133–34

  whole grains, 239

  See also Recommended Dietary Allowances (RDA)

Nutrients

  balance of, 37–38

  calories vs. ("A-" vs. "X-rated"), 22–23, 36, 217–20, 235–49, 285

  deficiencies in, and symptoms, 294–95, (tables) 297–334

  destroyed by light, 159

  in food vs. supplements, 44 *(see also* Dietary supplements)

  major, sources of (tables), 297–334

  measurement of, 295–96

  RDA of, *see* Recommended Dietary Allowances

  requirements (differences in), 7–8, 16, 23–24, 27, 28–29

  storage and loss of, 24–27, 38, 45, 85, 104, 126–27, 138, 139, 140, 253

Nutrients in Foods (Laveille, et al.), 190

Nutritional education, 39, 43

Nutrition Almanac (Kirschmann and Dunne), 190

Nuts and seeds, 38, 278, 281

  as cereal, 86, 88, 241

  and cholesterol, 264

  nutrient analysis (tables), 237, 241

  as oil/fat source, 216, 264, 265

  and peristalsis, 86, 87, 88

  roasted, and rancidity, 237, 241, 327

Oat products, 47, 87. *See also* Grains

Oils

  calorie content of, 141, 265

  cod-liver, 106, 140

  and constipation, 35, 86

  rancidity of, 140, 141, 237, 327

  sources of, 216, 265

  See also Fats; Salads and dressings

Osteoporosis, 125–27. *See also* Illness

Pantothenic acid: sources and deficiency symptoms (table), 321

Para-Aminobenzoic Acid (PABA): sources and deficiency symptoms (table), 332

Parratt, Dr.: quoted, 31

Pasta, 13, 261

Peristalsis, 69, 85–86, 88. *See also* Constipation

Pets, and relaxation of stress, 11

Phenylketonuria, 19

Phlegm, 45. *See also* Allergies

Phosphorus: sources and deficiency symptoms (table), 322. *See also* Minerals

Physical activity

  as adjunct to diet, 40, 188, 193–202, 204, 208, 287

  aerobic exercise, 206, 207–8, 258

  "belly bloppers" (for peristalsis), 87–88

  benefits from, 195–96, 279, 284

  calories burned by, 191, 193–201, 206, 214, 237–38, (tables) 191, 198–99

  cautions concerning, 197, 204, 207–8, 258

  choice of, 197, 200–202, 207–9, 212–13

  exercise with weights, 213, 214

  habits of, 205–6, 208–9, 284, 287

  and muscle weight, 212–13, 285

  running, 207, 213

"spot" exercises, 195–96
as stress response, 10–11, 214–15
walking, 200, 207, 208, 212, 215–16, 258, 284
Physician, consultation with, 294
before beginning diet, *xiv, xv,* 35, 36, 40, 50, 105, 124, 139, 174, 175
before beginning exercise program, 195
and diet supplements, 281
for medication change, 211, 278
and special problems, 235, 258
Pocket Diet, 36, 51, 157–72
Pollution, 42, 89, 104–5, 242, 265
Polyunsaturated fatty acids (PUFA), *see* Fatty acids, polyunsaturated
Potassium, 279
and constipation, 35, 85, 87, 88
-sodium balance, *see* Salt
sources, 86, 88, 140, 173, 227, 234, 258, 261
sources and deficiency symptoms (tables), 226, 323
storage and loss, 38, 45, 85, 128, 138, 139, 140
supplementary, 255, 281
See also High-Potassium Soup, Basic
Potatoes, *see* Vegetables, fresh
Poultry
and cholesterol, 107, 242
in diet, 38, 39, 219
fat/calorie content of, 140, 154, 242, 243, 262–67 *passim,* 278
hormone-treated, 20
Pregnancy, *see* Women
Preservatives, *see* Additives
Preserved food, *see* Processed food
Pressure cooker, *see* Cooking methods and equipment
Processed food, 236
canned or bottled (foods and juices), 45, 55, 129, 158, 160, 161, 170, 219, 255–60 *passim,* 265 (*see also* vacuum-packed, *below)*
cost of, 41, 269
fats/calories in, 22–23, 158, 218, 252, 262–69 *passim,* 335–36
labels on, 19, 129, 170, 219, 239, 250–56 *passim,* 260–61, 265, 266, 268–69
loss of food value in, 17, 23, 252, 255, 335–36
lunch meats, *see* Meats
in Pocket Diet, 36, 158, 170

refined, *see* Carbohydrates; Grains
sodium content table, 257
substances removed or added, 17–19, 45, 90, 158, 218, 252, 264, 268–69, 335–36 *(see also* Additives; Salt; Sugar)
vacuum-packed, 170, 237, 250, 269
Protein
allergies to, 45, 47
amino acids, 19, 334
deficiency of (in aging), 128
low-calorie diet and, 40, 179
men's need of, 82, 179
overconsumption of, 219
sources, 82, 179, 231, 232, 266
sources and deficiency symptoms (table), 324
See also High-Protein, Low-Carbohydrate Diet
Prunes, 70. *See also* Fruits, dried
PUFA (Polyunsaturated Fatty Acids), *see* Fatty acids, polyunsaturated
Pyridoxine, *see* Vitamin B-6

Quick High-Fiber Cereal (recipe), 242

Rabies, 28
Rancidity, 140, 141, 237, 269, 327
Raw Diet, 35, 51, 89–103, 159, 175, 227
Raw foods, 41, 250. *See also* Fruits, fresh; Raw Diet; Vegetables, fresh
RDA, *see* Recommended Dietary Allowances
RE (retinol equivalents), 291*n. See also* Vitamins
Recipes
Basic Grain Cereal, 240
Basic High-Potassium Soup, 228
Bone Stock, 232–33
Grain, Nut, and Seed Cereal, 241
Quick High-Fiber Cereal, 242
time-saving, 41–42, 227, 231 (*see also* Two-Minute Diet)
Recommended Dietary Allowances (National Academy of Sciences), 23, 289, 292
Recommended Dietary Allowances (RDA), 23–24, 37–38, 44, 49, 284, 286, 289–94
calcium, women and, 125–26
vs. dietary supplements, 41
met by additions to diets, 125, 169, 176, 179, 229

Recommended Dietary Allowances
(*cont.*)
nutrients for men and women (tables),
64–65, 291 (*see also* Nutrient
analysis)
Record-keeping, 36–37, 46, 52, 187,
204, 285, 286
calorie intake/output, 190–94, 197–
99, 201, 216–19, 249
negative and positive results, 67, 83,
102, 121, 136, 155, 171, 180,
189
sample record card, 191, 217
weight change, 68, 84, 103, 122, 137,
156, 172, 181
Refined foods, *see* Carbohydrates;
Grains; Processed food
Regularity Diet, 34–35, 51, 54, 69–88
Restaurant food, 11–13, 37, 45, 95,
218, 286
Riboflavin, *see* Vitamin B-2
Rice products, 48, 87, 237, 239, 261
allergy to, 47
See also Grains
Roasting process (nuts and seeds), 237,
241, 327
Roughage, *see* Fiber
Running, 207, 213. *See also* Physical ac-
tivity
Ryan, Dr. Edward J.: quoted, 19
Rye: allergy to, 47. *See also* Grains

Salads and dressings
bottled dressings, 260, 265
low- or no-calorie, 13, 230, 245–47,
265–66, 274
mayonnaise, 13, 38, 260, 266
Saliva
importance of, 182, 267, 280
lack of or thick, 125, 127, 128, 182
and salivary enzymes, 89, 280
See also Digestive problems; Teeth
and gums
Salt
elimination of, from diet, 44, 211,
227, 253–59
and fluid retention, 40, 211, 227,
249, 254, 256–59, 278
in processed foods, 45, 129, 158, 170,
218, 252, 255–56, 257, 266, 269
reaction to, 45, 106, 211, 253, 256–
57
sodium content of selected foods
(table), 257

sodium needs and overuse, 216, 256–
58, 293, 294
sodium-potassium balance, 40, 211,
237, 249, 253–55, 257–59
sodium sources (natural), 335
sodium sources and deficiency symptoms (table), 326
Saturated and unsaturated fats and oils,
see Fats; Fatty acids, polyunsatu-
rated; Oils
Saunas, 211, 258
Seafood, *see* Fish and shellfish
Seeds, *see* Nuts and seeds
Selenium: sources and deficiency symp-
toms (table), 325. *See also* Min-
erals
Senate Select Committee on Nutrition
and Human Needs (1977), 293
Shine (Anti-Stress) Diet, 35, 51, 104–
24, 280
Shopping for food, 10
and label-reading, *see* Processed food
Shopping lists, 49
High-Protein, Low-Carbohydrate
Diet, 142
Lean, Clean Machine Diet, 175
Pocket Diet, 160
Raw Diet, 91
Regularity Diet, 70–71
Shine (Anti-Stress) Diet, 108
Sweet Diet, 54–55
Two-Minute Diet, 129
Sleep
calories consumed during, 214
exercise and, 196
Smoke (in preserved food), 158. *See also*
Additives; Processed food
Snacks, 208–10, 268
Sodium-potassium balance, *see* Salt
Soil depletion or deficiency, 21–22, 253,
335
Soups and broths, 274, 281
as calcium source, 47, 105, 173, 231–
34 *passim*
canned, 45 (*see also* Processed food)
fat removed from, 38, 232, 234
thickening for, 235
as vegetable source, 43, 175, 229–30,
250–51, 274–75
water for, 227, 230, 232, 233,
250
See also Bone Stock; High-Nutrient
Soup; High-Potassium Soup,
Basic

Soybeans, 231, 250
  as calorie source, 276, 278
Spices, *see* Herbs and spices
Steaming, *see* Cooking methods and
    equipment
Stir-frying, *see* Cooking methods and
    equipment
Stress, *xvi*, 42, 125, 139, 158
  anti-stress diet, 35, 51, 104–24, 280
  eating/feeding as response to, 10–11,
    274
  illness as, 123
  and osteoporosis, 127
  physical activity as cause of, 207
  physical activity as relief of, 10–11,
    214–15
  See also Illness
Stroke, 39, 87, 253. *See also* Illness
Sucrose, 54. *See also* Sugar
Sugar, 216
  blackstrap molasses, 88
  low blood, 54
  overconsumption of, 27, 34, 44
  in processed food, 54, 129, 158, 218,
    252, 259–60, 269
  See also Carbohydrates; Sweet Diet
Sugar reserves (glycogen), 39–40
Sulfur: sources and deficiency symptoms
    (table), 334
Supplements, *see* Dietary Supplements
Suppositories, *see* Laxatives and suppo-
    sitories
Sweet Diet, 27, 34, 51, 53–68, 259

Taste preferences and dislikes, *see* Food
Teeth and gums, 280
  calcium loss and, 126, 127
  nutrient effect on, 35, 89, 182
  problems with, 90, 125–28 *passim*,
    175, 182, 234, 259, 267–68
  See also Digestive problems; Saliva
Temptations, *see* Food
Thiamin, *see* Vitamin B-1
Toxicity
  of additives, 18, 19, 20–21, 28, 45
  aluminum or lead, 170
  of dietary supplements, 28, 292
  of natural foods, *xii*, 18–19, 249
Tranquilizers
  calcium and magnesium as form of,
    28
  and diet restrictions, 21
Triglyceride level, 140
Two-Minute Diet, 39, 51, 125–37, 227

Veal, 242. *See also* Meats
Vegetables, canned, 129, 160
Vegetables, dried, 250. *See also* Legumes
Vegetables, fresh, 38
  cabbage family, 48, 235
  as calorie source, 243–44, 275, 276,
    278
  and cholesterol, 264
  and constipation, 86, 87, 140
  cooked vs. raw, 86, 90, 128, 175,
    182, 209–210, 227, 229–30
  high-carbohydrate, nutrient analysis
    (table), 238
  juices, 90, 175, 227, 230, 235, 249,
    251, 258, 274, 281
  low-carbohydrate, nutrient analysis
    (table), 243–44
  as mineral source, 86, 140, 281 *(see
    also* High-Potassium Foods)
  potatoes, 237, 238
  as roughage, 69, 86, 230
  vitamin content of, 236 *(see also* Vita-
    mins)
  See also Salads and dressings; Soups
    and broths
Vegetarian diet, 8, 34, 106, 264
Vitamin A, *xii*, 38, 192, 291*n*, 292
  sources, 106, 140, 236, (table)
    297
Vitamin B, 69, 266
Vitamin B-1 (thiamin), 101, 135, 169,
    179
  sources and deficiency symptoms
    (table), 298
Vitamin B-2 (riboflavin), sources and
    deficiency symptoms (table),
    299
Vitamin B-3 (niacin), 66, 82, 135
  sources and deficiency symptoms
    (table), 300
Vitamin B-6 (pyridoxine), 82, 135, 169,
    179
  sources and deficiency symptoms
    (table), 301
Vitamin B-12 (cobalamin), 174, 259
  sources and deficiency symptoms
    (table), 302
Vitamin C (ascorbic acid), 236, 251,
    281, 332, 335
  sources and deficiency symptoms
    (table), 304
Vitamin D, 106, 140, 292
  sources and deficiency symptoms
    (table), 310

Vitamin E, 17, 28, 135, 153, 174, 261
  sources and deficiency symptoms
      (table), 311
Vitamin K, 69
  sources and deficiency symptoms
      (table), 317
Vitamin P (bioflavonoids), 59
  sources and deficiency symptoms
      (table), 332
Vitamins
  excretion of, 24, 104
  RDA of, 64, (table) 291
  removed in processing, 269
  sources and deficiency symptoms
      (tables), 297–302, 304, 310, 311,
      317, 332
  supplemental, 44, 106, 281–82, 292
  See also individual vitamins

Walking, *see* Physical activity
Water
  bodily retention or loss of (fluid
      weight), 8, 34, 39–40, 211, 227,
      234, 249, 254, 256–59, 278–79
  content of, in food, 248–49
  used in cooking, 174, 227, 228, 230–
      35 *passim,* 240, 250
  See also Beverages
Weight
  fat, 211, 212, 234
  fluid, *see* Water
  muscle, 211, 212, 285
  "right," 210
  See also Weight gain; Weight loss
Weight change charts, *see* Record-
      keeping
"Weight faker," 211. *See also* Muscles
Weight gain
  diets or plans for, 34, 49, 190, 192,
      193, 210, 288
  food input level and, 201
  premenstrual, 278
  record-keeping for, 190, 192, 193
  size and frequency of meals and,
      25
Weight loss
  constipation and, 85

as criterion or priority in dieting, 23,
      34, 40
  diets for, 27, 39–42, 49, 138–39,
      174, 234, 244, 253, 288
  diets plus exercise for, 188, 204, 208,
      212, 215–16
  fluid loss and, 39–40, 211, 227
  muscle, 212
  need for, questioned, 6, 197
  "plateau" in program for, 273–75,
      278
  and record-keeping, 190–93
Weights, exercise with, *see* Physical ac-
      tivity
Wheat bran, *see* Fiber (roughage)
Wheat germ, *see* Grains
Wheat products
  allergies to, 47–48, 238, 239
  See also Breads; Flour; Grains
Whole grains, *see* Grains
Women
  B-12 deficiency in, 259
  and calcium loss, 125–26
  calories needed or burned by, 51, 66,
      126, 199
  diets unsuitable for, 36, 138, 139,
      153, 169, 179
  fluid retention by, 227, 258, 259, 278–
      79
  iron deficiency/need in, 38, 66, 82,
      101, 120, 135 169, 179, 291n
  muscle tone in, 213
  muscle weight loss for, 212
  and "plateaus" in weight loss, 278
  pregnant or lactating, 50, 139, 179,
      291n, 293
  RDA for, 64–65, 291
  running as exercise for, 207
  See also Menopause; Menstruation

Yams: calories in, 238
Yogurt, *see* Milk products

Zinc, 38, 45, 66, 153, 173
  sources and deficiency symptoms
      (table), 329
  See also Minerals